Lose Weight with Green Tea

A Safe Weight-Loss Method that Works

Patricia Rouner

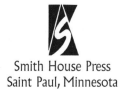

Smith House Press
Saint Paul, Minnesota

Smith House Press
P.O. Box 17948
Saint Paul, Minnesota
(651) 490-9408

www.SmithHousePress.com

Cataloging-In-Publication Data
Rouner, Patricia.
    Lose weight with green tea : a safe, sensible way toward weight loss management / Patricia Rouner.
        p. : ill. ; cm.
    Includes bibliographical references and index.
    ISBN: 0-9615221-7-8
1. Reducing diets. 2. Weight loss. 3. Green tea--Health aspects. I. Title.
RM222.2 .R68 2005
613.2/5

1 3 5 7 9 10 8 6 4 2

Cover by Mayapriya Long
BookWrights

To my aunt, Goldie Miller,
for her continual support
and her example of a well-lived life.

Table of Contents

Introduction 1

1. Green Tea and Weight Loss: The Science 9

2. From Tea Bush to Teacup:
   Growing and Processing Tea 19

3. Never Use Boiling Water:
   The Right Way to Brew Green Tea 35

4. Have You Hugged Your Polyphenols Today? 53

5. If It's Tuesday, Is Caffeine Okay? 59

6. Extracts: Can I Just Take A Pill? 71

7. It Fights Disease, Too 83

8. What's Right For You? 99

Appendix A: Other Weight Loss Suggestions 109

Appendix B: Reuse and Recycle 115

Appendix C: Resources 121

Appendix D: Glossary of Terms 139

Index 145

Acknowledgments

Every book is a team effort, both in front of and behind the computer screen. Steve, Stephanie and Kiera deserve thanks for traversing piles and piles of papers and books without injury and without comment (at least within my hearing range). A special thanks to my son, Patrick, who, in addition to the above, kept the tea cupboard full and the teakettle hot.

Thanks also to my favorite uncle, Merle Miller, for continuing to be.

Special thanks to my sister, Verlene, who helped beyond measure when needed.

Bill Waddington, the Tea Guy, was incredibly nice and very patient to a rookie tea drinker. His knowledge and love of tea provided energy to the book and his TeaSource stores provided sustenance.

Thanks to Beth Upton for her enthusiasm, insightful comments and great abilities in fine tuning the manuscript, and to Mayapriya Long for her amazing cover design abilities.

Finally, she-who-has-no-asterisk, the amazing Sybil Smith, friend and publisher, I thank you for your patience, your confidence, your care and concern and, most of all, your wacky sense of humor.

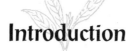

Introduction

*Curb your appetite! ***
*Speed up your fat burning! ***
*Lose weight and not be hungry! ***
*Lose ten pounds in five days! ***
*Forget calories! Forget carbs! ***

The claims are enticing. When I see them on television or in a magazine or newspaper ad, it's sometimes tempting to think that just by taking a pill or a few capsules a day I could lose those extra pounds. The ads often imply I won't have to give up my favorite foods and won't even have to look at a treadmill. Better yet, some ads hint that I can lose weight while sleeping. I could deal with that. But then I see the asterisk.

There's always an asterisk. It's usually quite small and easy to miss. The asterisks after the claims refer to additional information that can be found in the ad, usually at the bottom in very small type. They're almost always accompanied by the words "When used with our diet and exercise program" or a similar statement. Darn.

Sometimes the ads show a beautiful woman who tells us that she lost 20 pounds while still eating all the chocolate she wanted. She too has an asterisk somewhere or a disclaimer that runs quickly along the bottom of the screen and says, "Results not typical." Double darn, especially since sometimes the "before" and "after" photos seem to imply that while losing the weight your teeth will be whiter and straighter, your hair will look thicker and shinier and somehow, despite the weight loss, your bust size will increase. It's especially intriguing when the woman is at least two inches taller in the "after" picture.

So when a friend claimed she had lost several pounds without changing her diet, but simply by drinking green tea, I was skeptical to say the least. I looked her up and down but couldn't find the asterisk. I did notice she had indeed lost weight; she looked better and seemed to have more energy. Over the next few weeks we had some meals together and I could see her appetite hadn't diminished, nor had her helpings; she ate like she wasn't dieting. I could also see that she had lost even more weight. I asked more questions about green tea and her answers intrigued me enough to do some research.

The more I researched the more interested I got. Green tea had not been part of my vocabulary, much less my diet. My whole life has been spent with coffee drinkers. When I was a child coffee was an occasional treat in which to dunk a cinnamon roll. Like so many, I started drinking coffee on a regular basis in college. Tea was something I saw only in a Chinese restaurant or politely sipped when nothing else was offered at a friend's house. I tried herbal teas once in a while after reading their health benefits, but always preferred coffee. I even went to a formal afternoon tea at a restaurant with friends, but have to admit I enjoyed the sandwiches, the scones and the ceremony more than the tea.

The last several years I have had a small box of Earl Grey tea on hand because I knew some friends preferred it, but I didn't know there was such a thing as green tea, much less oolong, white or red tea. Through my research I have been introduced to a tea world I didn't know existed. I have found it to be fascinating, surprising and amazingly promising—fascinating because of the history and traditions associated with tea, surprising because of the findings of the many studies I read, and promising because the ongoing research indicates we are getting closer to finding the answers for many of the health issues we face today, including obesity. Green tea may be an important component of those answers.

Let me be clear. I am not an expert. I'm a writer and editor who has edited enough medical books and articles to have a pretty good medical vocabulary and a really good chance at spelling words correctly. More important, I have a library of medical reference books and if I'm not totally sure of a term, I'll find it and keep reading until I understand it.

It's harder to figure out which reports are true and which ones are guesses or opinions, what research is flawed, or who has a vested interest in the results, i.e., a cereal company sponsoring research with results saying cereal is good for you. There's a lot of research being done, sometimes with conflicting results, and those results can take years to sort out. As we have seen, there is still much we don't know about nutrition, disease, and medicine; most important, there is much we don't know about the human body and its interaction with nutrition, disease and medicine.

The Internet has made researching any issue so much easier, so much more productive and so much more confusing. When you find the information, you have to judge whether the site is reliable enough to count on the accuracy of the information. I've tried to do that. I'll discuss the importance of research in Chapter Eight, because after all that I've learned in the last few months, I'm convinced each of us must become an MD—a "Me" Doctor.

One answer I wanted to find out was pretty basic: how many people in the United States are overweight? We are constantly hearing that we're an overweight society and, frankly, I had tuned it out. When I read the statistics, I was shocked. When I started to really look at other people, especially groups of people, I had to admit the statistics are correct. Almost two-thirds of adults in the United States are overweight.

I was one of them. Having been thin most of my life I hadn't given it much thought. Even after I gave birth to two children, weight wasn't an issue, though I'll admit my fitness level wasn't great. I got into the routine of collapsing on the couch in front of the television when the children were finally asleep. But then, as the years went by, I noticed the dreaded "middle-age spread" was attacking and vowed to do something about it right after…I completed the editing job I was working on…the holidays…as soon as the birthday cake was gone ("Wouldn't want to waste good food")… Monday, okay, maybe next Monday. I don't know why I thought I had to start on a Monday. But that's the way it went for too many holidays, too many birthdays, and way too many Mondays.

Middle-age spread is a reality and can start when we're in our 20s. Without changing our eating habits, we slowly gain about a pound per year. Women tend to store fat in their hips and thighs until menopause and then the fat shifts somewhat and thickens the waist. Men gain weight in a somewhat similar fashion, resulting the infamous "beer belly."

We all know how to lose weight: burn more calories than you take in. That's not always easy and, given the statistics, rarely done, especially as we get older. And it's not your imagination that it's harder to lose the pounds as you get older. Our metabolism slows as we age so it takes more energy to burn those calories.

That brings us to green tea and why it can help us lose weight. The short answer: it speeds up metabolism and helps our bodies burn fat, about 80 calories a day. The result: if you're in your 40s, 50s, or older, drinking green tea may help you lose the pounds that have crept up on you. If you're in your 20s or 30s, you may be able to prevent middle-age spread with the help of green tea. If you're heading for college, you could ward off the notorious "Freshman 15," the fifteen pounds many students gain during their first year of college.

A caveat (or an asterisk): If you're extremely overweight or obese, you're not going to lose all of those pounds simply with green tea. But green tea can give an added boost to your weight-loss efforts. It has been used safely for centuries, it's reasonably inexpensive, it provides nutrients without adding calories or artificial chemicals and it has far less caffeine than coffee or colas.

Caffeine is constantly in the news. Is it good or bad? We'll look at both possibilities in Chapter Five. We'll also look at an easy way you can decaffeinate tea in your own kitchen.

First, though, we'll look at the 1999 research study that created the interest in green tea, and some of the other studies that have corroborated those findings. Then we'll take a quick walk through some of the world's tea gardens to learn how tea is grown and processed. All tea comes from the same plant; it's the processing that determines whether it will end up in your cup as a dark, bold, wake-me-up black tea, a soothing green tea or a delicate white tea.

America was a tea-drinking nation until that little incident in Boston in 1773 known as the Boston Tea Party. It's taken more than two centuries but Americans are again learning to enjoy tea. For those not familiar with brewing tea (as I was not) we'll talk about the two most important ingredients, the tea and the water, in Chapter Three. We'll also discuss how to choose and store tea and the various methods of brewing. Hint: green tea should not be brewed the same way you would brew black tea.

Chapter Four will explain why researchers think green tea can help us lose weight. Then we'll figure out what antioxidants are and why we need them, as well as why we don't want free radicals.

You may have seen ads for extracts of green tea. Can you just take a pill and lose weight? Chapter Six will look at the pros and cons.

There is far more research about the other health-related benefits of drinking tea. Though this book is primarily about the weight-loss aspects of tea, we should be aware of what science is saying about its disease-prevention possibilities. Chapter Seven will go over some of that research, including the asterisks.

In the back of the book you'll find other tips on losing weight, how to deal with tea stains, and recycling ideas for tea and teabags, as well as resources to learn even more about tea. But first we'll answer the burning question: how much tea do you need to drink to lose weight or ward off disease? Chapter Eight will answer that question as well as get you started on becoming your own MD ("Me" Doctor). It will also tell you what kinds of information you can and cannot expect to get from your colleague, the one with the medical degree on the wall.

Chapter One

Green Tea and Weight Loss: The Science

Though the many benefits of green tea have been known in Asian cultures for centuries, most research on tea by Western scientists didn't begin until the mid-1980s. Research is by nature time-consuming and expensive, with many false starts and dead ends. Some research projects take years, publishing the results can take many months and follow-up research can stretch into decades. By Western scientific measure, research on green tea is in its infancy.

The first mention of tea as an aid to losing weight was recorded centuries ago by the Chinese, usually referring to Pu-erh tea. Studies published in the mid-80s garnered a little attention, but it wasn't until the late 1990s that Western scientists started to look seriously at green tea.

The University of Geneva Study

A 1999 article published in the *American Society for Clinical Nutrition* began to generate interest in green tea as a possible aid in losing weight. Though tea has been widely consumed throughout the world for centuries, little scientific study had been reported on its effects in humans. A team of scientists from the University of Geneva (Switzerland), interested in plant ingredients that might affect weight loss in humans, wanted to see if the caffeine and catechin polyphenols (natural compounds in green tea) would make a difference in the energy expenditure (metabolism) and fat oxidation (fat burning) in humans. Since the Geneva study was the major catalyst for interest in green tea and continues to generate additional studies, let's look at how the research was done and what was learned.

Researchers recruited ten healthy men who were classified as lean to mildly obese (8–30% body fat) to participate in the research study. They did not include anyone who smoked, who was a competitive athlete or who had a history of weight loss. They wanted men who regularly consumed a typical Western diet, one with fat contributing 35–40% of dietary energy. Each man's physical characteristics were noted, including height, weight and percentage of body fat.

On three separate occasions each subject spent 24 hours in a respiratory chamber. They were randomly assigned one of three treatments: 1) two capsules of green tea extract which contained 50 mg of caffeine and 90 mg of epigallocatechin gallate (EGCG), a powerful antioxidant found in tea leaves, as well as other ingredients naturally found in green tea; 2) two placebo capsules filled with cellulose, which has no effect on the body; or 3) two capsules with 50 mg of caffeine. The caffeine capsules contained no additional ingredients.

The dietary energy intake (number of calories) and diet composition for each man were identical and were categorized as weight-maintenance. The food-energy content was about 13% protein, 40% fat and 47% carbohydrates. No other foods or drinks with caffeine were allowed for 24 hours before or during the time in the respiratory chamber. The men's sedentary lifestyles, physical activity, meal patterns and sleep times were similar during the testing periods. The men read, watched television or listened to the radio while in the respiratory chamber. They did not exercise. There were three 24-hour testing periods for each man over a period of 5–6 weeks.

The Results

Using respiratory and urinary testing, the scientists found that the men who had been given the green tea capsules had a four-percent increase in energy expenditure in 24 hours. Caffeine is known to affect metabolism but in this study the caffeine alone had no effect on the subjects, perhaps because the dosage wasn't high enough to stimulate metabolism. The subjects who got the caffeine capsules consumed a total of 100 mg of caffeine at each meal, less than the caffeine in an average cup of brewed coffee. The same amount of caffeine was in the green tea capsules but the caffeine was not responsible for the increased metabolic effects. The scientists speculated that the caffeine and the components of the green tea, working together, caused the increased metabolism and fat oxidation. What is not known is whether green tea that has been decaffeinated would have as much of an effect on metabolism and fat oxidation. More about caffeine and its effects on humans can be found in Chapter Five.

The scientists also learned that the men given the capsules that contained green tea extract and caffeine did not experience increased heart rates, making it a safer alternative than other drugs used to help lose weight, especially in people with high blood pressure or other cardiovascular problems.

So, to simplify and translate, the men who got the green tea capsules burned an extra 80 or so calories in a 24-hour period without exercising and without changing their normal diets.

Other studies

Another study reported in the online edition of the January 2005 *American Journal of Physiology: Regulatory, Integrative and Comparative Physiology* showed that mice that had been given green tea extract over a ten-week period showed increased exercise endurance of 8-24% more than mice that exercised but were not given the extract. What's more, they found the mice given the extract burned fat more efficiently. Scientists reduced the amount of caffeine in the extract for the experiments and concluded that caffeine was not a factor in the increased endurance and fat oxidation. Additional experiments found that the catechin epigallocatechin gallate (EGCG), a polyphenolic (antioxidant) compound found in green tea, improved endurance, though the evidence was weak, suggesting that the other catechins in green tea were also necessary.

A single dose was not effective in increasing metabolism, leading to the conclusion that long-term use of green tea was necessary to replicate the results. It should be noted that the research was done at the Biological Sciences Laboratories of Kao Corporation in Tochigi, Japan, which makes health care products, including green tea beverages. That doesn't mean the results were skewed, but is mentioned in the interest of full disclosure.

Researchers in another study, published in the journal *Phytomedicine* in January of 2002, confirmed that green tea extracts did not increase heart rates during weight loss. Seventy moderately obese subjects were given two green tea extract capsules daily, containing 270 mg of EGCG, one-third more than in the

University of Geneva study. The results after three months: body weights decreased by a mean of 4.6% and waist circumferences by 4.48%.

A 12-week Japanese study on the effects of catechins on body fat reduction involved men of similar size (based on body mass index, an indicator of fat, and their waist circumferences) who were given different amounts of catechins. One group was given tea fortified with green tea extract that contained 690 mg of catechins, while the other group was given tea that had only 22 mg of catechins. During the three-month test the men ate identical breakfasts and dinners and were told to control their calorie and fat intake at other times so that overall diets were similar. At the end of the 12 weeks, waist circumference, body weight and body mass index were all significantly lower in the men who were given the tea containing the green tea extract. The men in that group lost an average of 5.3 pounds versus an average weight loss of 2.9 pounds for the other group.

A Chinese test was done on 75 people who were considered to be obese due to overeating and/or lack of physical exercise. The people, between the ages of 22 and 69, were asked to drink oolong tea twice a day for six weeks. They were asked to eat normally, not to try to diet, and to refrain from exercising.

Using echography sensors to measure the thickness of subcutaneous fat near their navels before and after the six weeks, researchers found an average decrease of four millimeters. In addition, the tests showed serum, total cholesterol and serum triglyceride levels were lower after the six-week test. Sixty-seven percent of the participants lost weight during the testing. Remember, they had no dietary guidelines and there was no documentation of what they ate during the testing period.

Another study done in Taiwan studied the tea-drinking habits of 1,103 people and analyzed body fat differences and waist-to-hip ratios. Results: those who had been drinking tea for more than ten years had 19.6% less body fat on average and 2.1% smaller waist-to-hip ratios than those who did not regularly drink tea. They concluded that tea could be a weight-loss beverage.

As I mentioned earlier, the scientific study of tea as a weight-loss mechanism is in its infancy. More information is published almost daily, and much more research is on-going.

Other studies have also shown green tea's efficacy in burning fat and increasing metabolism but far more studies have been done on the cardiovascular benefits of tea and tea's disease-fighting capabilities. Chapter Seven will go over some of what has been discovered.

Frequently Asked Questions

What are nutraceuticals? Is green tea considered to be a nutraceutical?

Sometimes referred to as functional foods or phytochemicals, nutraceuticals are foods, parts of foods or derivatives of foods—natural chemical compounds—that have health benefits, either in preventing or treating disease. The interest in nutraceuticals has grown as some scientists have turned their attention to foods as a complement or possibly an alternative to pharmaceuticals. Chicken soup for colds and beta-carotenes are examples of nutraceuticals. Green tea is considered a nutraceutical, as are all teas.

How many calories are in a cup of green tea?

Green tea itself has no calories, no sodium, no carbohydrates and no protein. Adding flavorings, honey for example, will add calories, of course.

How long does tea's metabolic action last?

One study looked only at the tea catechins to determine absorption levels and the length of time they stay in the body. They determined that after 8 hours over 90% had been excreted, which indicates that continual drinking of tea is necessary to keep the fat burning and metabolism stimulated. In addition, there is some indication that the catechins seem to encourage enzyme activity that may also promote weight loss.

Chapter Two

From Tea Bush to Teacup: Growing and Processing Tea

Legend says that sometime around 2727 BC, Emperor Shen Nung was resting near a small cauldron of boiling water when a breeze blew leaves from a nearby tea plant into the water. The aroma is said to have intrigued the emperor, who bravely drank the fragrant water and discovered the drink we now know as tea. Whether the story is true or not, tea has continued to intrigue people through the centuries and is second only to water in popularity around the globe.

All tea comes from the *Camellia sinensis* plant, which grows in over 50 countries, including China, Japan, Sri Lanka, India, Indonesia, Argentina, Kenya, Taiwan, Bangladesh, Uganda, Malawi, Turkey, Iran, Brazil, Australia and Tanzania. In general, the further the country is from the equator, the less tea is grown there.

Today there are over 3,000 varieties of tea grown in thousands of tea gardens and tea estates, sometimes called tea plantations. The unique characteristics of the different teas result from soil conditions, temperature, rainfall and even the altitude at which the tea is grown. Does that remind you of what is said about the grapes grown for wine? Tea is often named for the region in which it is grown, just like wine. And just as grapes can produce different flavors from year to year depending on the amount of rain, the condition of the soil, etc., so too can the quality and taste of tea leaves vary.

Even the descriptions of the various types and flavors of tea are much like those for different wines: delicate, grassy, nutty, malty, woodsy, fruity, full-bodied, smoky aftertones. And as with wines, there are various "grades," from very basic to extremely fine (read: cheap to very expensive).

Tea is a perennial shrub and sprouts new growth continually except in parts of India, China, Iran, Turkey and other areas where seasonal climate changes cause dormancy for a short period of time each year. Further from the equator, dormancy periods are longer.

Warm, humid climates that have an annual rainfall of at least 70 inches are generally required for growing tea. Most tea plants prefer deep, well-drained soil that is light and acidic. While some varieties of tea grow well at sea level, the premium teas prefer the cool mountain mist of the higher altitudes (up to almost 7,000 feet above sea level). Tea leaves grown in the cooler temperatures and higher altitudes are often considered to have superior flavor because the leaves develop more slowly.

The Tea Plant

The tropical evergreen tea shrub has a rough, gray bark and shiny dark green leaves. If allowed to grow wild, the evergreen shrubs would grow up to 30 feet tall, but they are usually kept pruned to three or four feet when the harvesting is done by hand-plucking. To make them a little easier to pluck, tea plants are pruned to have a flat top called a plucking plateau or plucking table.

On more mechanized farms, the plants may be allowed to grow as tall as seven feet. They are usually planted 40-60 inches apart in rows about 40 inches apart. Four thousand to six thousand bushes can be planted per acre, depending on the topography.

A tea bush may produce good tea leaves for 50-70 years, though there are claims of 80-year-old and even older bushes that are still going strong. Young bushes are grown from cuttings and take from three to seven years to come to maturity; it varies depending on the climate and conditions.

Some tea is grown on farms called smallholdings, which are only slightly larger than an acre. Other larger tea estates, which can be hundreds of acres in size, often resemble small communities. Some are so large they have housing, schools and even hospitals for employees and their families.

Harvesting (Picking or Plucking)

For centuries, tea leaves have been harvested by hand, usually by women because they have the fine motor control and dexterity to pick the delicate leaves and buds without damaging them. For premium teas, only the top two leaves and leaf buds are plucked, or picked, from each plant stem.

Tea picking, or plucking, is tough, hard work. The women endure heat and humidity, and often work on the sides of mountains, which makes their work especially difficult. Imagine trying to keep your balance on a steep hillside while the sun is beating down on you and insects are buzzing in your ears as you work quickly to pluck leaves. Then imagine doing so with a large basket on your back. That's how much of the world's tea leaves are harvested. A skilled worker can fill her basket with almost 70 pounds of leaves in a day.

Where tea grows throughout the year it is harvested every 7-14 days. Plants closer to sea level provide new growth much faster than those at higher altitudes because of the cooler temperatures at the higher levels. In cooler regions there are two prime picking times for quality teas. The first leaves of the new growing season, called first flush, are picked in the early spring and usually have a more delicate flavor than the second flush leaves, which are plucked in early summer, and are appreciated for their bolder flavors.

Hand-plucking is the only way most quality teas are harvested but shearing and mechanized harvesting are also done in many regions to harvest much of the world's tea. Some tea estates use hedge-clipper type shears, while in Australia machines similar to large lawn mowers are used to cut off new growth, harvesting almost 9,000 pounds per hour. Because machines cannot be as careful or accurate as hand-pickers, machine-harvested tea often contains unwanted stalks and older leaves, resulting in teas of inferior quality.

A good acre-yield for hand-plucked tea is between 200 and 500 pounds, while machine-plucked yields can be as high as 600 to 800 pounds per acre. In round numbers, it takes 100 lbs. of tea leaves to make 20 pounds of tea, but that amount can vary depending on the size of the leaves and any additions made to the tea leaves for flavoring.

Geography, growing conditions and the soil account for the differences in the tea leaves, but the processing of the leaves is what determines if the tea will be black, oolong, green or white.

Processing the tea leaves

Once the tea has been plucked it is taken to a factory to be processed. In an area of small farms the tea is processed by a factory that is centrally located among a group of smallholdings—much like corn is taken to centrally located co-op elevators in the Midwest of the United States. On larger estates, this is usually done at an in-house processing factory.

The traditional or orthodox method requires more hands-on ministrations and today only the best leaves are totally hand processed. Hand processing increases the cost of the tea but some find that the quality of flavor is so superior it is worth the extra cost. For green tea, the leaves are first dried by putting them in withering bins or spreading them out on concrete, bamboo or woven straw racks in the sunlight or with warm air circulating around them to evaporate any moisture. The oxygen changes the colors of the leaves and enhances their flavors. Timing is critical.

Depending on the country and the type of tea desired, the oxidation is stopped by quickly steaming or pan-frying the leaves. The heat prevents the oxidation of polyphenols, the chemical substances that provide antioxidant protection against disease, but it maintains the potency of the flavonols, the chemical compounds that give tea its unique flavor.

In China, higher-end teas are put into large woks where they are tossed, turned and carefully tended until they are evenly dried and flaccid. Flowers are often added during the drying process when scents are desired. Jasmine, chrysanthemums, orange blossoms, cherry blossoms and roses are some of the flowers used.

The leaves are then rolled and shaped to release essential oils. The method differs depending on the country, culture and tradition but in some countries the rolling and shaping method is considered part science and part art.

The leaves finish drying, then they are sorted or graded. The leaves are sorted by leaf size using wire mesh. The larger leaves are used for loose-leaf tea while the smaller particles, sometimes call tea dust or fannings, are used for teabags because they can be quickly brewed.

This is a simplistic description of the growing and processing of tea and only minimally reflects the scientific art of tea processing that has evolved throughout the centuries. If you're interesting in learning more about how the methods differ from country to country, even from province to province, there are several books that go into detail. A list of books about tea and tea processing can be found on pages 121–122.

Pu-erh Tea

While most tea is processed and marketed as quickly as possible to take advantage of its freshness, Pu-erh tea is aged for 30 years or more before being consumed. Little known in the West until recently, the tea comes from the Yunnan Province in southwestern China and has been used by the Chinese for centuries to relieve stomach upsets, lower cholesterol and aid in weight loss.

Older tea leaves from old tea plants are used for Pu-erh tea. They are fermented for three months or more, which allows bacteria to enter the leaves. Some leaves are left loose while others are formed into bricks or cakes. They are then buried for many years and allowed to age.

Pu-erh may turn out to be the tea healthiest for humans but it is described as having a "strong, earthy, complicated," taste. One source describes Pu-erh as an "acquired" taste.

Frequently Asked Questions

How is black tea processed?

Black tea undergoes further processing and oxidation is allowed to continue until the leaves turn a golden brown or black. A method called CTC (crush, tear, curl) is often used to literally tear the leaves apart, allowing faster oxidation. The oxidation gives black tea its characteristic robust, more full-bodied flavor.

What is oolong tea?

Oolong, the tea common in Chinese restaurants, is oxidized for one to two hours, half the time of black tea, before it is heated. Since oolong is oxidized less than black tea (but more than green tea), it has a milder flavor than black tea.

Are herbal teas similar to green tea?

Not really. Herbal teas are not really teas, since only leaves from the *Camellia sinensis* plant can truly be called tea. A beverage made from herbs is a tisane (pronounced tih-ZAN). Tisanes have been used for medicinal purposes for centuries.

Does tea tree oil come from the tea plant?

No. Tea tree oil, which is often used to treat cuts, stings, insect bites, athlete's foot, and many other injuries and conditions, comes from the Australian *Melaleuca alternifolia* tree and has no relationship with tea plants.

Is tea grown anywhere in the United States?

Surprisingly, yes. On an island twenty miles from South Carolina's shore, the Charleston Tea Gardens have produced American Classic tea since 1987. The only tea producer in the U.S., the 127-acre Charleston Tea Gardens is located on Wadmalaw Island where tea is harvested from May through October. Tours are available. Check their web site, www. charlestontea.com for more information.

What is red tea?

The term "red tea" can be confusing because it is the name the Chinese use for what we know as black tea. But today when someone refers to red tea, they usually mean Rooibos (pronounced Royboss), or red bush tea, which is becoming better known in the United States. Rooibos is technically not a tea and does not come from a red bush. It comes from the *Aspalathus linearis* plant and has needle-like green leaves that turn red during processing, thus the name. It has gained much popularity in the U.S. during the last few years because of its sweet, slightly nutty taste. Grown only in South Africa, Rooibos has no caffeine and is a rich source of vitamins and minerals so it is considered to be a healthy drink for pregnant women and nursing mothers and even for colicky infants. Rooibos is often used to treat allergies and skin irritations. In Japan it is known as long-life tea.

What is white tea?

White tea is tea that has been processed even less than green tea. The leaves for white tea are carefully plucked before the buds open. They are then withered to evaporate the moisture and dried without allowing oxidation. White tea requires intensive hand processing so it is a bit more expensive. It may be an even healthier drink than green tea but very little research has been done to determine this for sure. White tea should be brewed with water at a lower temperature (170 degrees), never with boiling water. The flavor is very light and slightly sweet and it contains the least caffeine of all teas. Chapter Five talks more about caffeine.

What country produces the most tea?

Though China is the country most people first think of when talking about tea, India actually produces the most tea, about one-third of the world's tea, two billion pounds. China, Sri Lanka, Kenya and Ceylon follow in amounts of tea produced.

If there's such a difference in teas, why does my favorite tea always taste the same?

Since the weather and other growing conditions can affect the taste of teas, tea manufacturers use a blend of teas to ensure that favorite teas taste the same every time the consumer brews them. Professional tea tasters sample dozens or even hundreds of tea each day from different regions, estates, even seasons, to determine the amount needed from each to make the "standard," familiar tea that ends up in your cup.

Should I be concerned about pesticides in tea?

That's difficult to answer. Because tea has natural enemies, herbicides and pesticides are used to thwart them. Some countries use more chemicals than others, but many are trying to use more natural methods and fewer pesticides.

Are there organic teas?

Yes, and more are being produced all the time, but it's not simply a matter of deciding to "go organic." For many tea growers it means a total change from the use of fertilizers, pesticides, or chemicals of any kind anywhere on the estates. Only natural methods of pest control, such as using pest-eating insects, are allowed.

Pesticides can stay in soil for years so the soil must be rejuvenated, which means not growing tea there for some time, not something many tea growers can afford to do. Also, many contaminants are still allowed to pollute the air throughout the world and those contaminants can be carried with the wind or come down in rainfall.

There are organizations that inspect, monitor and certify organic products. If you want to make sure you're using an organic tea, look for the organic certification symbol on the package.

Are people who work on tea estates treated well and fairly?

In relative terms (the average wage of the country), tea workers have traditionally been paid fairly well. Concerns about the changes in the tea industry, especially those involving tea workers in developing countries and the buying-up of tea estates by large conglomerates, have resulted in some companies agreeing to the strict economic, social and environmental auditing by Fair Trade associations.

Fair Trade is a collaboration between tea pickers, tea distributors and tea drinkers that assures fair wages, decent living conditions and reasonable working conditions for the pickers. A percentage of every tea purchase is guaranteed to go back to the workers. Usually a committee of workers then decides what is most needed by the community, for example, better health facilities, electricity or more teachers.

TransFair USA is the certifying organization in the United States. Look for the Fair Trade label on tea packages if you want to be sure you're buying tea from a Fair Trade company.

Tea Trivia

The tradition of leaving tips was started in the tea gardens of England. Tip boxes were left on the tables with the sign: "To Insure Prompt Service"—TIPS.

When tea was first introduced to England it was quite expensive; milk, however, was cheap. It is said that the amount of tea added to milk was an indication of social standing. The wealthy drank the tea without milk. The middle class added some milk to their tea and the lower classes added a little tea to their milk.

By World War II tea was so important to the British that stocks of tea were hidden in 500 places all over England to guard against the air raids of the Luftwaffe destroying the tea supply.

Chapter Three

Never Use Boiling Water: The Right Way to Brew Green Tea

If, when you think of drinking tea, you think only of pretty teapots, china teacups and flowery chintzes, please be assured that if that's not your style, there is another tea world, one of heavy stoneware mugs, Thermoses and even plastic water bottles...and everything in between. Brewing and drinking green tea can be adapted to anyone's lifestyle and can provide a healthy beverage to drink all day long.

Yes, there are tea connoisseurs who will be appalled by some of the ideas in this chapter, but what is important is getting the weight loss and health benefits of the tea. If you don't have a teakettle, you can boil water in a saucepan. If you prefer teabags to loose tea leaves, fine. What is right for you is what is right. Period.

The most critical factors in brewing tea are the water, the temperature of the water and the tea. We'll go over each in detail.

Water

Water is the most important part of brewing tea. Though the United States arguably has the safest tap water in the world, it's not always the best tasting. If your water doesn't taste good, your tea will not taste good. There are many types of filters for tap water, ranging from expensive whole-house filters, to under-sink filters and filters that attach to your kitchen faucet.

There are also pitchers that use replaceable filters. Just fill the reservoir with tap water and in a few minutes the water will taste cleaner and fresher. The newer models make it easier to know when the filters need replacing.

The filters usually remove most of the chlorine, lead and copper in the water. The lead and copper can be from the water pipes in your home, so it's especially important to use a filter if you have an older plumbing system, not just for making tea but for your own health and especially the health of any children living in the house. The filters may also remove fluoride from your water, which could be a concern if you have small children. Talk to your pediatrician or pediatric dentist about how much fluoride your children need to prevent tooth decay and about other sources of fluoride.

If your area has hard water, the calcium in it can cause tea to be murky and it can affect the taste. Though chlorine can be boiled out of water, over-boiling the water will affect its taste and the taste of the tea. Filtering your water is often an easier way to get rid of the unwanted chemicals.

Household water filters are not meant to remove all of the impurities that can be found in well water but the filters can improve the taste. If you have a well, have your well water tested regularly for safety.

Reverse osmosis, also known as hyperfiltration, is probably the most effective water treatment. It can produce water that is 99+% pure. Household units are commercially available.

Some consider spring water to be the best water with which to make tea because of its mineral content and the lack of additives, such as chlorine, that are usually found in tap water. But if you choose to buy spring water make sure the bottle says it is spring water; if it is labeled "drinking water," it could be just filtered tap water, something you could produce yourself with the filters mentioned above.

The minerals in water are necessary for good-tasting tea, so never use distilled water (which has had all minerals removed). It will produce a tea that tastes very flat and does not offer the nutritional benefits of the minerals.

Once you've found the water that tastes best to you, it's time to choose your tea.

Teabags: An Accidental Dunking

In the early 1900s, samples of different teas were often left by tea merchants for restaurateurs to taste-test before they ordered large amounts for their restaurants. The different teas were encased in small silk bags. One restaurant owner is said to have inadvertently dunked a bag of tea into hot water and discovered he could have the taste of tea without having to deal with the leaves swimming around in his cup. Soon tea merchants were experimenting with all types of papers and fabrics to find the best method to contain the tea but allow its flavor to escape into the cup. Americans, even at the turn of the last century, were willing to give up some of the tea flavor in favor of convenience.

Choosing tea

There is such a wide variety of green teas on the market that it's fun to purchase a few kinds and try them to see what you like and don't like. Even if it turns out that you don't like the flavor of one or more kinds, they won't go to waste. Green tea has a mild enough taste that by adding a flavorful tisane (herbal "tea") to your cup you can modify the taste of the tea to your liking while still reaping its benefits. Or you can add spices like cloves and cinnamon to adjust the taste to your satisfaction. For additional flavors, consider adding lemon, herbs, mints, licorice, Rooibos, ginger, or any flavor that appeals. You can even add fresh fruits (mango, melon balls, strawberries, pineapple—it's up to you) or fruit juice and have a tea sangria. Just remember that if you're trying to lose weight, fruits and fruit juice are sugar, albeit more nutritious than the white stuff.

If you're new to tea and lucky enough to have a tea merchant nearby, ask for recommendations. Stores are popping up throughout the country, offering a wide selection of teas from all over the world. The store-owners are often extremely knowledgeable about their teas and can help you decide what to try first. Also, more restaurants are offering afternoon "teas." If you can, take advantage of one or more. A variety of teas are offered for you to try and the food is usually great, an added bonus.

The first decision you have to make is whether you want to use teabags or loose-leaf tea. Tea lovers will insist that only loose-leaf tea should ever be used, but the convenience of teabags is making them popular even in Great Britain. And, of course, you can choose to have both. Many of the boxed teas offered in your local supermarkets are fine to drink, even if they contain slightly fewer polyphenols than loose tea.

When buying loose-leaf tea, look at its color. The tea leaves should be a dark, rich green, though some varieties are more of a gray-green. Again, rely on your tea merchant for help. Sometimes they will even offer taste samples.

Testing the tea for aroma is another way to determine freshness. If there's little or none, it's probably too old. If it smells pleasant and sweet, even grassy, it should be okay.

To test the freshness of your box of teabags, take the tea leaves out of one teabag and pour hot water over the empty bag. If the water tastes like water, the teabags are fresh. If the water tastes like tea, the tea has been in the bag too long.

Storing tea

Once you've brought your tea home it must be stored correctly to retain its flavors. Light, moisture and other odors are the main enemies of tea. Tea should be stored in an air-tight opaque container. The container should be just large enough for the tea; if too little tea is stored in too large a container, it will continue to oxidize. If you are keeping your tea in a foil bag be sure to squeeze as much air out as possible when you take out tea and make sure it is sealed tightly. Glass and ceramic are good materials for storing tea. Never store tea in clear glass because light alone will cause loss of flavor and freshness.

Don't store tea with other spices. Tea will pick up any odors near it.

Storing it in a refrigerator makes tea vulnerable to odors and moisture, but if you're confident of your packaging and have a small refrigerator to use exclusively for tea, with temperatures between 30 and 40 degrees Fahrenheit, tea can be stored for six months.

Tea can be frozen, but only if you're extremely confident of your packaging. If you can't freeze meat without it suffering from freezer burn, don't try to freeze tea.

Don't open your container of dry tea leaves near your boiling teakettle. The humidity in the air can affect the rest of the tea. Also, make sure any utensil you put into the tea container is totally dry. A drop of water left in the container will change the taste of the remaining tea leaves.

To be on the safe side, it may be best to buy only 2–4 ounces of tea at a time. That may not seem like a lot but one ounce should provide 15–30 cups of brewed tea, so it's more than one would expect. Part of the secret of getting so much brewed tea from so little dried leaf is that the tea leaves can be used over and over. You can expect three or more cups of tea from one teaspoon of tea leaves. Teabags, too, can be used again and again. The taste will be somewhat different with each cup, but still pleasant.

Smaller leaves often weigh more than larger leaves, so fewer leaves are needed. If possible, use a small food scale or postage scale to weigh the tea rather than using a teaspoon of leaves. First use the recommended amount. You will soon learn how much to use to suit your tastes and will be able to judge the right amount by sight alone.

Brewing the tea

If you're new to brewing tea, expect to make some mistakes. The water may be too hot or not hot enough. You may steep (soak) the tea too long or not long enough. Each time you make tea you will learn a little more about what you like and don't like. Pretty soon you'll love every cup.

Water temperature

Water temperature is critical to the taste of your tea. While black tea needs boiling water (212 degrees), green tea abhors boiling water and will quickly turn bitter. Err on the side of cooler, rather than hotter. That goes for teabags as well as loose tea. Sometimes the manufacturers use the same instructions on their boxes of black teas and green teas. Ignore any instructions that tell you to pour boiling water on your green tea and consider changing brands.

For green tea the water temperature should be between 160–175 degrees Fahrenheit. There are differing opinions among the experts as to whether the water should be heated just to the correct temperature or heated to boiling, then cooled to the correct temperature. Try it both ways and see if it makes a difference to you. But if you have any questions at all about your water supply, boil it first, then let it cool. The easiest way to test the temperature of the water is to use a candy thermometer. A candy thermometer can be found for five dollars and will help until you're able to judge the water temperature yourself.

Another method is to heat the water to just boiling, then add cool water to lower the temperature. Splashes could be dangerous so be careful, and don't use this method in a delicate china cup; it could crack or break.

If you're using a teakettle, there are several ways to judge the temperature of the water. If you have a whistling teakettle, listen for the first tentative tweets. That will be about the right temperature for green tea. A shrieking teakettle, of course, means the water is boiling. If you have the time to watch the teakettle, take off the whistler and watch the steam come out of the spout. Steam that wafts back and forth means the water is right for tea that requires a lower temperature (like a white tea). When it starts to shoot straight out, take the teakettle off the heat; it's ready for most green tea. NOTE: If you have teenagers, make sure they know why you're staring at the steam. Even then, they may wonder about you.

If you don't have a teakettle you can use a saucepan to boil the water. When tiny bubbles begin to appear in the water, take it off the heat. Just be careful of splashes. There are also electric teakettles and other appliances that will heat the water to precise temperatures.

Steeping

While the water is heating, prepare your teapot or cup. It's good to heat the pot or cup by putting hot or boiling water in it, then emptying it. This helps to keep the tea warm longer. Add the teabag(s) or the loose tea. Loose tea can be added directly to the teapot or cup, or it can be put into a type of infuser which should be large enough to corral the tea leaves and still allow the expansion or unfurling of the tea leaves. There are many other kinds of strainers, including bamboo infusers. Some teapots have built-in strainers to do the job. Metal tea balls are also available but they are often too small to allow the leaves to fully expand.

You can make your own teabags. Several kinds of disposable or reusable bags are available for purchase in tea shoppes or on the Internet. You add your own tea leaves and brew as usual. Using these bags provides the convenience of a bag and allows you to make sure there is enough room in the bag for the leaves to expand. Try to find bags that are unbleached, without added chlorine.

When the water is ready, pour it over the tea leaves or teabags. Let the green tea steep for the length of time recommended on the box or bag, usually for one to three minutes, though it's really up to you. Experiment and find the right time length for the flavor you like. High-quality green tea should be pale green to yellow green when properly brewed, but other ingredients in the tea (lemon, flowers, etc.) may influence the color.

Remove the teabag or infuser and allow the tea to cool to drinking temperature. If you've used loose tea leaves, they should have all sunk to the bottom of the cup by the time the tea is cool enough to drink.

The Brits Get More

British teabags are generally larger than American teabags (allowing for better tea expansion) and many think that the tea in British teabags is a better quality of tea because the manufacturers believe the British have more discerning tastes in tea. Perhaps in the next few years, U.S. tea drinkers will demand what their British cousins already enjoy.

Other methods of brewing

If you like using loose tea leaves but don't like them floating in your brewed tea, try using a tea press. Similar to a coffee press, the plunger pushes the leaves to the bottom, allowing you to pour the leaf-less tea into your cup.

You can also use a coffeemaker, though it may not heat the water hot enough. Thoroughly clean any coffee residue from the coffeemaker, then measure tea leaves into a coffee filter, add the water and brew as you would coffee. If this works for you, you may want to buy a separate coffeemaker to be used only for tea.

Microwaving the water to brew tea is frowned upon by many and done every day by many more. If you know your microwave and learn to judge the temperature of the water, and the tea tastes good, then do it. But be aware that microwave ovens vary widely; some may not be able to boil water while others can superheat the water, making it dangerous to remove the cup from the oven. To be on the safe side, let the cup sit for a minute before trying to remove it. A candy thermometer can again be of help in judging the temperature of the water.

Whatever method you use, heat fresh water for that second or third cup of tea. Remember, re-boiled water lacks oxygen and will be flat or have a metallic flavor.

Heat + Ice = Iced Tea

The 1904 St. Louis Exposition was held during a people-wilting heat spell and no one was interested in the vendor's hot tea. Frustration being the father of invention, the desperate vendor asked to borrow some ice from a nearby ice cream vendor. He added ice to a cup of hot tea and offered the new cool drink to the crowds. Lines began to form and iced tea has been the most popular tea drink in the United States for over 100 years.

Remember

The most important part of brewing tea is finding out what you like. Break the rules, experiment, make mistakes; just find out the best way to drink one of the healthiest drinks on earth: green tea the way YOU like it.

Iced tea

Iced tea makes up almost 85% of the tea consumed in the United States. Available in almost every restaurant, it is not just a summertime favorite, but popular throughout the year.

To make your own iced tea, brew your favorite tea but double the number of bags or amount of tea leaves. Fill a pitcher two-thirds full of ice (made from spring or filtered water, of course). Remove the teabags or strain the tea, then pour the hot tea over the ice. Add more ice until the tea is diluted to twice its initial volume. Or use 1/8 cup of tea leaves in a coffee maker basket and add water to brew 12 cups or the full capacity of the coffeemaker. Add water to dilute to taste.

If you have time, brew tea regular-strength, fill an ice cube tray with the tea and freeze. When you want iced tea, put the frozen tea cubes in a pitcher, then fill the pitcher with regular-strength brewed tea. You won't have to worry about the tea being too diluted when the ice cubes melt. Enjoy!

A word about sun tea. Sun tea is made by adding teabags and water to a clear jar and leaving it in direct sunlight for a few hours. Though fun to make and delicious, it apparently doesn't get warm enough to release the polyphenols, though there is some question about this.

Frequently Asked Questions

I don't have a way to heat water for tea at work. Are there any good ways to transport tea to and from work?

Probably the easiest and best way to transport either hot or cold tea is with a glass-lined steel vacuum flask (Thermos). The larger ones can hold several cups of tea. Just make the tea in the morning and it will stay quite warm most of the day. If you can't find a glass-lined flask or don't want to use one (the glass can break) you can use a metal-lined flask but you may find there is a metallic taste to your tea. To avoid this you can build a patina on the inside of the flask. Brew several cups of strong tea and pour it into the flask. Leave the tea in the flask for several hours. Do not wash the flask after you do this. Just add your tea every day and drink as usual. Soon you'll find there is no metallic taste. One important note: If you do this, do not drink directly from the flask as that would introduce bacteria.

A friend of mine carries her tea wherever she goes in a plastic water bottle. I've heard that plastic water bottles are dangerous. True?

This is a common misconception...maybe. I had read the same thing, even in reputable magazines. When I researched the question I learned that the answer is a bit complicated. There were some e-mails going around that said you should never freeze plastic water bottles because dioxin in the bottles would be released. Another story was about a grade school where kids' water bottles were found to be loaded with bacteria.

The dioxin rumor was false. There are no dioxins in plastic water bottles. Dioxin is produced only when plastics are burned.

As for the bacteria in the kids' water bottles, it turned out they had been refilling them day after day for weeks without taking them home to be washed. Kids being kids, all kinds of nasty bacteria were introduced to the bottles from mouths and hands and started growing to dangerous levels.

You should wash your polycarbonate (Nalgene is the most popular brand) or other plastic bottles frequently with soap and water but never in the dishwasher. The intensity of the dishwasher detergent can cause minute bits of plastic to slough off into any liquid introduced to the bottle.

The lighter-weight plastic bottles used for most over-the-counter water can be used a few times but then should be recycled. Since they were manufactured for single-use, they have never been tested for refilling or multiple uses.

Chapter Four

Have You Hugged Your Polyphenols Today?

Though they don't choose to use the term "nutraceutical," Steven Pratt, M.D., and Kathy Matthews, in their popular book, *SuperFoods Rx*, list tea, both black and green, as one of 14 foods that are so nutrient-dense they can improve your well being and help you live longer. The other "super foods" (in alphabetical order) are beans, blueberries, broccoli, oats, oranges, pumpkin, salmon, soy, spinach, tomatoes, turkey, walnuts and yogurt. These super foods (including tea), according to Pratt and Matthews, are all foods high in micronutrients and phytonutrients. Micronutrients include vitamins and minerals while phytonutrients are other substances that provide valuable health benefits. In 2002, *Time* magazine published a similar list of ten foods. Most of the food items were the same with the marvelous additions of garlic (because of its allyl sulfides, which can reduce cholesterol) and red wine (for its polyphenols, of course).

Phytonutrients

Green tea provides micronutrients and an abundance of phytonutrients, especially polyphenols. One type of polyphenol, flavonoids, are also found in red wine (there's the wine connection again) and berries. A subclass of flavonoids, flavanols, includes catechins, theaflavins, thearubigins and proanthocyanidins. Just to add more confusion, another class of flavonoids, flavonols (notice the "o" instead of the "a"), is also found in tea. While catechins are affected by the processing, thus are more abundant in green and white tea (green tea has 4–5 times more catechins than black tea), flavonols are less affected by the processing and can be found in both black and green tea. They are mentioned because there are hints that as more research is completed and published, black tea, which also contains the catechins theaflavins and thearubigins, may be found to provide health benefits similar to green tea and may even prove to be more beneficial in certain cases.

Most of the research on the health benefits attributed to green tea has been focused on the catechins as being primarily responsible. Catechins are found in tea, chocolate, grapes, berries and apples. The principal catechins found in tea are epicatechin (EC), epigallocatechin (EGC), epicatechin gallate (ECG) and the star of the show, the one getting the most attention, epigallocatechin gallate, or EGCG. One cup of freshly brewed green tea (8 oz) can provide anywhere from 5 to 200+ mg EGCG. The amounts differ depending on where the tea has been grown, the growing conditions, when it was picked, how it was processed and how it is brewed. The more catechins the better. Catechins have antioxidant powers that are stronger than vitamins A, E and, according to the results of one test, almost 20 times stronger than vitamin C and possibly even stronger.

Antioxidants

So what, exactly, is an antioxidant? We all know the value of oxygen and how much we need it. We also know it can be damaging (think rust or freezer-burned meat). In our bodies, when oxygen interacts with certain molecules, oxidants called free radicals are formed. Free radicals can cause damage to our cells, even to our DNA, and can cause cells to function poorly or even die. Cigarette smoke, too much sunlight, radiation, pesticides, etc., can also produce free radicals. Our bodies provide several enzyme systems to battle the dastardly free radicals, but additional troops arrive in the form of antioxidants. Antioxidants that are not formed within the body must be supplied through our diet in the form of fruits, vegetables or dietary supplements.

Vitamins E (nuts, seeds, vegetable and fish oils, apricots, fortified cereal, whole grains) and C (citrus fruits, green peppers, cabbage, spinach, broccoli, kale, cantaloupe, kiwi, strawberries) and beta-carotene (liver, egg yolk, milk, butter, spinach, carrots, squash, broccoli, yams, tomatoes, cantaloupe, peaches, whole grains), which is converted to Vitamin A in our bodies, are high in antioxidants. Now we know WHY we're supposed to eat five servings a day of fruits and vegetables. And why we need green tea.

And from the nothing-is-ever-easy department: For some reason, exercise, which increases our need for oxygen, also increases free radicals. This is called exercise-induced free radical damage. However, experimental studies have shown that regular physical exercise helps our own natural systems to battle the increased free radicals. Some doctors recommend increasing antioxidants, such as by drinking green tea, before and after exercising. The operative word, though, is "regular" exercise. It takes some time for our bodies to balance out the exercise-induced free radicals and the body's natural defenses. People who tend to exercise only on the weekends are not allowing their bodies to provide that balance.

It should be noted that free radicals are not all bad. For example, they are used by our white blood cells to destroy bacteria and virus-infected cells. Some chemotherapy treatments rely on free radicals to kill cancer cells and antioxidants could interfere with the effectiveness of the cancer treatment. The body is complicated and the diseases that attack it are also complicated. If you are fighting cancer, be sure to discuss the value of antioxidants with your oncologist.

Frequently Asked Questions

Can't I get all my nutrients, including antioxidants, from food?

That depends, of course, on your diet. But it also depends on how well your body absorbs the nutrients (stress and age can affect absorption). More important is how nutritious your food is. Where, when and how your food is grown all make a difference in the quantity and quality of the nutrients in the food.

I like milk and sugar in my tea. Do they affect the flavonoids?

Most people do not use milk or sugar in green tea the way they do in black tea because the taste of green tea is much milder. If you do want to use them, they will not affect the effectiveness of the flavonoids, despite what some web sites say. Of course, they will affect the calorie count. If you're trying to lose weight with green tea, forget the milk and sugar, but if you're drinking tea for its other health benefits, which will be discussed in Chapter Seven, drink it any way you like.

Some Green Teas and Their Antioxidant Levels

	EGCG (Mg/100 ml)	Total catechins (Mg/100 ml)
Celestial Seasonings Green Tea	99.3±1.8	216.2±0.5
Lipton Green Tea	83.9±2.8	196.6±5.2
Uncle Lee's Green Tea	65.0±7.1	155.7±13.2
Salada Green Tea (Earl Green)	49.8±3.6	108.5±8.6
Salada Green Tea Decaf	46.3±0.7	86.8±0.7
Bigelow Green Tea	42.5±2.5	87.5±4.6
Celestial Seasonings Green Tea Decaf	37.7±0.8	72.3±0.7
Stash Premium Green Tea Decaf	20.7±1.8	52.7±5.0

Source: Henning, Susanne M., et al. "Catechin content of 18 teas and a green tea extract supplement correlates with the antioxidant capacity" 2003. *Nutrition and Cancer* 45(2), 226-235.

While this is interesting, it was only one test and there is no definitive answer as to why there was such disparity. Subsequent tests with different lot numbers of tea (teas harvested at another time) may produce different results.

Chapter Five

If It's Tuesday,
Is Caffeine Okay?

It's so confusing. One morning you open a news-paper and read that caffeine is dangerous for everyone. By that evening, the network anchor is telling you caffeine can help athletes increase their performance and a new study says children with ADHD are more focused when they have...guess what? Caffeine. How do you know what to believe? More important, what's best for YOU?

Nine out of 10 Americans use caffeine from some source on a regular basis. Depending on your attitude, caffeine may be the most abused drug in the world, a necessity to help you face the morning, or one of the four basic food groups (the latter attitude is often found among college students at mid-term time).

Caffeine is a slightly bitter alkaloid, known medi-cally as trimethylxanthine, and is found in seeds, leaves, or fruits of more than 60 plant species grown worldwide. Though it occurs naturally in some plants, caffeine is added to many other foods, drinks and drugs. Coca-Cola adds caffeine to its products "for flavor purposes only." Barq's Root Beer has a "bite" that is attributed to the caffeine that has been added to it. Products like Excedrin and Anacin contain added caffeine because it increases their effectiveness, sometimes by almost 40 percent.

Caffeine is probably the most studied drug in history, but even though much is known about it and how it affects the human body, there is still much to learn. Let's look at what is known: the good, the bad, and the ugly.

The good:

- Caffeine wakes you up, mentally and physically. It can increase alertness for several hours.

- It can start to work its magic in as little as five minutes (especially in coffee).

- It improves muscle coordination and strength when consumed immediately before exercise. Note: It is one of the substances not allowed by the International Olympic Committee.

- To a very small extent, it helps burn calories.

- It is thought that caffeine helps to relax the airways in the lungs and may be associated with fewer asthmatic attacks in those who have asthma.

- It may lower the incidence of Parkinson's disease.

- In men, it may decrease the formation of gall-stones.

- It can act as a laxative (that could be good, bad or ugly).

- It can dampen your appetite, but only temporarily.

- It acts as a mild stimulant on the kidneys and digestive organs.

- In combination with other drugs, caffeine eases migraine headaches.

- It increases the power of aspirin and other pain relievers. One study even concluded that caffeine by itself was as effective as acetaminophen (Tylenol) for non-migraine headaches.

- In women suffering from PMS, caffeine, which is a diuretic, can decrease bloat.

The bad:

- It may increase the risk of osteoporosis in women, especially if they are drinking coffee or tea instead of drinking milk.

- It raises blood pressure slightly, but only temporarily.

- It is addictive. Do you think soft drink manufacturers add caffeine to their products just for the flavor?

- Contrary to popular belief, caffeine does not help a hangover.

- Caffeine can impact some medications. Ask your pharmacist if drinking tea will impact the effectiveness of your prescriptions.

- Some women report caffeine increases breast tenderness but, in spite of earlier reports, there is no link between caffeine and breast cancer (as of this writing).

- It can cause a temporary fall in blood sugar.

- It can irritate the bladder.

- It can cause increased anxiety.

- Caffeine can increase the production of stomach acid and affect the valve between the esophagus and the stomach, causing acid reflux and heartburn. This may occur even with decaffeinated tea or coffee.

- Consuming caffeine in the evening, sometimes even in the afternoon, can cause some people to have trouble falling asleep at night.

- It can cause slight hand tremors, which can be a problem depending upon your profession or hobbies.

The ugly:

- Some studies indicate caffeine may cause miscarriages when four or more cups of coffee (450+mg) are regularly consumed. It also has been shown to slow the growth of a developing fetus and may also affect the heart rhythm of a fetus.

- Caffeine can pass into breast milk and be a stimulant for a nursing infant.

  Even doctors who are not particularly concerned about the normal effects of caffeine caution pregnant and nursing mothers to reduce or abstain from all caffeine.

Sensitivity

The vast majority of people tolerate a moderate amount (300 mg) of caffeine very well, but there is a wide range of sensitivity to caffeine. Sensitivity to caffeine depends on a number of factors but includes:

- body mass. The smaller you are the less caffeine you need to feel its effects, both bad and good;

- the amount of normal caffeine use. If you don't use caffeine on a regular basis, it will have a stronger effect when you do; and

- stress. Both psychological stress and physical stress (such as heat stress) can increase your sensitivity to caffeine.

Those who drink or eat more than 500–600 mg of caffeine per day may find it causes restlessness, anxiety, headaches, nausea and other gastrointestinal distress and irritability.

Some people are ultrasensitive to caffeine. Even a morning cup of tea or coffee can keep them awake at bedtime and the caffeine's effects can last into the next day. And there are people who are allergic to caffeine, though the numbers are controversial.

In addition, it's not easy to know how much caffeine you're ingesting. While companies are required to list caffeine as an ingredient if it is added to a product, they don't have to list the amount on the label or can. For example, even though kola nuts contain a natural amount of caffeine, Coca-Cola is required to list caffeine on the label only when more caffeine is added to their products. However, nothing on the can or bottle will tell you how much caffeine is in the drink. I was surprised to learn Diet Coke has quite a bit more caffeine than Coca-Cola Classic.

The following list gives a general idea of how much caffeine is in various products.

Double espresso (2 oz)	45–100 mg
Brewed coffee (8 oz)	60–120 mg
Ben & Jerry's Coffee Fudge Frozen Yogurt (8 oz)	85 mg
Jolt (12 oz can)	71 mg
Instant coffee (8 oz)	70 mg
Excedrin	65 mg
Mountain Dew (12 oz)	55 mg
Mello Yello	52 mg
Diet Coke (12 oz)	46 mg
TAB	46 mg
Dr Pepper	41 mg
Pepsi Cola (12 oz)	36 mg
Coca Cola (12 oz can)	34 mg
Vanquish	33 mg
Anacin	32 mg
Midol	32 mg
Nestea Sweet Iced Tea	26 mg
Baking Chocolate (1 oz)	26 mg
Snapple Green Tea w/Lemon	24 mg
Barq's Root Beer (12 oz)	22 mg
Dark chocolate (1 oz)	20 mg
Tea—black (8 oz)	**23–110 mg**
Tea—oolong (8 oz)	**12–55 mg**
Tea—green (8 oz)	**8–36 mg**
Tea—white (8 oz)	**6–25 mg**
Milk chocolate (1 oz)	6 mg
Chocolate milk (8 oz)	4 mg
Decaffeinated coffee (8 oz)	1–5 mg
Decaffeinated tea	**1–4 mg**

The answer to whether or not you should drink beverages with caffeine, or how much to drink, is found inside you. If you think you need to cut back on caffeine, or if your doctor has suggested it, do it slowly and carefully. Depending on your normal intake of caffeine, abrupt withdrawal can cause severe headaches, fatigue, irritability and nervousness that can last up to a week.

To cut back on caffeine safely, first try to determine how much caffeine you're getting in your regular diet. Don't forget to count the caffeine in chocolate and the hidden caffeine in various medications. Then gradually reduce your caffeine until you're feeling comfortable. If you're a coffee drinker, tea can be your answer.

Caffeine in tea

The amount of caffeine in a cup of tea is determined by a number of factors including where the tea is grown, the soil conditions and the altitude. Even the location of the leaf on the tea plant makes a difference.

Tea preparation has the most effect on caffeine. The size of the tea leaf, the temperature of the water and how long the tea is steeped in the water all make a difference. For example, black tea infused for 5 minutes contains 40–100 mg of caffeine, depending on the other factors, but if infused for only 3 minutes, the caffeine in the tea is only half as much. Since teabags often contain the smallest particles of tea leaves, which easily release their components, more caffeine is produced. Green tea is brewed at a lower temperature so a cup of green tea contains less caffeine. The brewing of tea is discussed in Chapter Three.

The caffeine in tea is absorbed more slowly than the caffeine in coffee. Instead of the 5 minutes it takes to feel the effects of your morning coffee, it takes almost 20 minutes before the caffeine in tea wakes you, but the gentle effects of the caffeine in tea last longer than the quick coffee jolt.

If you're ultrasensitive to caffeine or simply want to be as caffeine-free as possible, try decaffeinated tea. As you could see on page 65, decaffeinated tea has the least amount of caffeine of any of the products listed.

How tea is decaffeinated

There are two methods of decaffeination allowed in the United States, ethyl acetate and carbon dioxide. Ethyl acetate is often referred to as "natural" because its components are found in some plants, including bananas, coffee and tea leaves, but it is a strong solvent that requires warnings on its packaging and caution in its use. As the ethyl acetate passes through the tea leaves the caffeine bonds to it and is eliminated with the ethyl acetate. Unfortunately, this method also carries away almost 70% of the catechins, the beneficial ingredients in tea.

A better method, one that preserves almost 95% of the catechins and leaves no toxic residue, uses carbon dioxide. At high temperatures under pressure, carbon dioxide becomes both a gas and a liquid. To decaffeinate tea, carbon dioxide is pumped into the chamber containing the tea leaves. The caffeine molecules attach to the liquid carbon dioxide and are pumped out together. The carbon dioxide process is more expensive but is being used more and more as its health-related benefits are recognized.

Either method removes about 97–98% of the caffeine from tea. Many tea manufacturers explain on their web sites which method is used for their products. If you can't find it, call and ask. Contact information is required to be on the tea packaging.

Decaffeinate your own tea

You can decaffeinate your tea in your own kitchen simply by steeping your tea for 30–45 seconds in hot water, then throwing away the water (or let it cool, then feed it to your houseplants—see page 111). Refill your cup with more hot or boiling water (depending on the kind of tea) and let it steep as you usually would. This method removes 80% of the caffeine, but almost no flavor or aroma will be lost.

Frequently asked questions:

I've been told that tea actually has more caffeine than coffee. Can that be true?

Pound for pound, tea has more caffeine. In other words, a pound of tea leaves has more caffeine than a pound of coffee. But a pound of tea leaves will produce about 300 cups of tea, while a pound of coffee yields only 80 cups.

Is the caffeine in tea the same as the caffeine in coffee?

Yes, though in 1827, when it was first extracted from tea leaves, it was thought to be different and was called "theine." When science showed it was not a different substance, theine became caffeine.

Are flavonoids lost in the decaffeinating of tea?

Yes. Decaffeinated tea can lose more than half of its flavonoids during the decaffein-ation process, depending upon which method of decaffeination is used.

I thought caffeine was supposed to be bad for every-body. What happened?

Early in the twentieth century it was thought to be a serious problem but it is now getting a second look. Remember how eggs were a no-no for many years? In case you haven't kept up, eggs are now considered to be a good source of protein, with limited effect on human cholesterol levels. If "Do unto others..." is the golden rule, "Moderation in all things" should probably be the "silver rule."

Chapter Six

Extracts:
Can I Just Take a Pill?

In most of the studies described in Chapter One, the subjects were given capsules of green tea extracts. The extracts had standardized amounts of catechins, or compounds of multiple substances that were carefully measured so the researchers were assured that each person or animal was given the same amount of the same kind of tea extract.

A recent UCLA study led by Dr. Susanne M. Henning tested the absorption of antioxidants in 30 volunteers to find out whether drinking tea or taking a supplement provided the most benefit. After the volunteers were given green tea, black tea or green tea extract, several blood tests were taken over a period of 8 hours. They found that the participants who received the extracts absorbed more flavonols, which led to a "small but significant" increase in antioxidant levels in their blood.

If you're not in one of the research studies, can you get the antioxidants provided by green tea in supplements instead of by drinking tea? Yes and maybe. Green tea extracts are available everywhere, in discount stores, pharmacies, grocery stores and, of course, over the Internet. They're available in capsules, liquids, powders, patches and even chewing gum.

The problem is the quality of the supplements. What is in them varies and it's not always apparent what you're buying. Some tea extracts contain caffeine (in varying amounts depending on the brand) while others are decaffeinated. Many supplements labeled as green tea contain other ingredients that are not necessarily familiar and are sometimes questionable.

Therefore, although it is sometimes easier and more convenient to swallow a capsule than to brew a cup of tea, it's not always easy to know which of the supplements in the marketplace will give you the benefits that a cup of tea offers. Some will give you more extracted flavonoids in one capsule than you could drink in several cups of tea; others may simply be filled with tea leaf fannings (tea dust left over from the processing) in far smaller amounts than what is contained in a tea bag.

Supplements

Since scientists don't absolutely, positively know for sure what ingredients or what combination of ingredients in green tea provide the health benefits, there is some concern that a capsule made up of only some of the green tea compounds may not contain the mixture of nutrients and phytochemicals necessary for full effect. A 2002 article in *Time* magazine listed green tea as one of ten foods that may prevent disease. The article quotes JoAnn Manson, chief of preventive medicine at Harvard's Brigham and Women's Hospital, as saying, "It may be the combination of antioxidants, phytochemicals and fiber that work together to confer health benefits." Manufacturers of supplements make up their own combinations of ingredients; the amounts of each ingredient will differ among the brands too.

One large discount retailer sells a brand of green tea extract that is clearly labeled as having standardized ingredients, 300 mg of green tea including 150 mg of polyphenols. A national nutrition chain store sells a bottle of green tea extracts (315 mg) that contains only 44 mg of polyphenols. It's less expensive per capsule, but you have to take almost four capsules to get the same amount of polyphenols. One brand, purchased at another discount retailer, says in big letters that it is a Green Tea Diet supplement. The back of the box talks about the University of Geneva study but the "Supplement Facts" state there are only 100 mg of green tea extract and polyphenols are not mentioned at all. Still another brand claims to have 90 mg EGCG in each capsule, but both of the last two brands also have 250 mg of chromium, a trace element you may or may not want or need. So look carefully at the labels to see which have the ingredients you're looking for in the amounts you feel are safe for you.

WARNING: With tea as with so much else, there is growing evidence that there can be too much of a good thing. High doses of antioxidants may not only NOT help, but may be dangerous. Large doses of beta-carotene have been shown to **increase** the risk of lung cancer in male smokers. And a recent (2005) University of Mississippi study, published in the *Journal of Natural Products*, found evidence that extremely high doses of green tea extract may harm, rather than help. Yu-Dong Zhou, a molecular biologist at the University of Mississippi's National Center for Natural Products Research and the lead researcher in the study said, "Drinking green tea still is good for you...There are thousands of years of evidence on that, but the idea of taking the equivalent of hundreds of cups of tea a day is something that needs to be looked at carefully." They found that instead of shutting down the mechanisms that help certain tumors survive and grow, the high doses may activate them. In their research they also found that epigallocatechin (EGC) in the tea had different effects depending on the type of tumor.

Dan Nagle, an associate professor of pharmacognosy in the University of Mississippi School of Pharmacy, who also worked on the study, pointed out that

"Nearly all the evidence of the beneficial effects of green tea comes from studies on populations who consume green tea, not tea extract in the form of powder, concentrates or pills." Needless to say, much more research needs to be done. In the meantime, common sense and moderation are still good guides.

If you choose to use green tea supplements, or any other types of dietary supplements, make sure you mention it to your doctor or do the research to know that the supplements won't interact negatively with any prescription or over-the-counter drugs you may be taking. For example, if you're taking Coumadin, which is a blood thinner, you should be aware that ginkgo biloba, aspirin and vitamin E can also thin the blood, so taking any combination of that drug and supplements could cause excessive bleeding. That would be especially important for doctors to know if you should need surgery. Green tea, too, is a blood thinner to a small extent because of the Vitamin K it contains.

FDA Regulations

A *USA Today* story on green tea extracts said the supplements are in the government's sights: "We are aware that green tea extract has become more popular in weight-loss supplements and that the promotional literature touts it as a metabolism booster," said Richard Cleland, an attorney with the Federal Trade Commission. "At this point, the publicly available evidence is not adequate to demonstrate that green tea extract will have a profound effect on metabolism or cause substantial weight loss." The article goes on to say the FTC won't say it's investigating any of the claims or advertising for this product.

That's not surprising, because the Dietary Supplement Health and Education Act (DSHEA) of 1994, signed by President Bill Clinton, says that the Food and Drug Administration (FDA) does not need to approve dietary supplements before they are delivered to the marketplace. Before 1994, dietary supplements were under the same regulations as other foods, but since the enactment of the DSHEA, only "new" dietary ingredients are subject to governmental scrutiny. A new dietary supplement is one that meets the definition of a dietary supplement but was not sold in the United States before October 15, 1994. However, there is no authoritative list of ingredients that were marketed before October 15, 1994, so the manufacturers and distributors decide whether an ingredient is new or not.

The manufacturers and distributors are also the ones responsible for ensuring that their labels are accurate. The list of ingredients and "supplement facts" on the labels are supposed to match what is in the bottle or box, but there is no oversight to assure that all manufacturers and distributors comply. FDA regulations require a label to have a descriptive name (like "Green Tea Extract") and it must say "Dietary Supplement."

The label needs a complete list of the ingredients in the supplement, the nutrition information, called "Supplement Facts," and the net contents of the product. The manufacturer's or distributor's contact information must also be on the label.

A dietary supplement is defined as a product taken by mouth that contains a "dietary ingredient" intended to supplement the diet. This could include any number of vitamins, minerals, herbs, amino acids, enzymes, organ tissues, glandular tissues and metabolites.

The manufacturer or distributor of the dietary supplement is also responsible for determining the safety of the supplement, for adequately substantiating any claims or representations made about the product and for ensuring no claims are false or misleading. But there is little or no oversight of those claims. The FDA does not even keep a list of manufacturers and distributors.

From the U.S. Food and Drug Administration: "By law (DSHEA), the manufacturer is responsible for ensuring that its dietary supplement products are safe before they are marketed. Unlike drug products that must be proven safe and effective for their intended use before marketing, there are no provisions in the law for FDA to 'approve' dietary supplements for safety and effectiveness before they reach the consumer. Also unlike drug products, manufacturers and distributors of dietary supplements are not currently required by law to record, investigate or forward to FDA any reports they receive of injuries or illnesses that may be related to the use of their products. Under DSHEA, once the product is marketed, FDA has the responsibility for showing that a dietary supplement is 'unsafe' before it can take action to restrict the product's use or removal from the marketplace."

In 2004, ten years after the DSHEA went into effect, the FDA announced it was beginning to look at making additional changes to its policies and procedures, but as of now the DSHEA is still in effect. So do not think because a supplement is on a store shelf or can easily be bought over the Internet that the government has declared it to be safe and effective.

Choosing a Supplement

When choosing a supplement, look at the label carefully. Look for what is there and what is not there. Some labels will tell you the percentage of polyphenols in each capsule, and some will even tell you the number of milligrams of EGCG, while others simply say they contain green tea extract. Some have warning labels saying that no one under 18 should take the supplements; others say no one under 12, and still others make no statement about age.

If you can't tell whether or not a supplement contains what you are looking for, contact the manufacturer and ask questions. Ask about the evidence that their product does what is claimed on the box. Ask if any tests have been done on the safety and effectiveness of the product. Does the company have a quality control system in place to make sure that what is on the label is actually in the capsule? In the case of green tea as well as many herbal products, can they assure you that pesticides or other contaminants in the supplements don't exceed safe levels? Also ask if they've received any reports of adverse effects from their products. Don't accept anecdotal evidence from "satisfied customers" and remember that charts and graphs are easy to do on any computer.

If you're researching a supplement or thinking of buying from a company on the Internet, look at who is running the site. Is it a government, university, hospital or medical association, or is it a company marketing its products? Obviously a company is not going to publish negative information about its product.

See if you can determine the purpose of the site. Many supplement manufacturers and distributors have done a good job of masquerading as informational sites. It's not until you've read the information (propaganda in some cases) that they try to sell you their products.

Also check to see whether or not the site is kept up-to-date. One reputable hospital's site has a ton of information on green tea, none of it newer than 1995, even though they are currently running clinical trials on the effects of green tea.

Frequently Asked Questions

Is black tea as healthy for us as green tea?

There is some thought that the oxidation process of turning tea leaves into black tea destroys many of the phytochemicals. But even though almost 80% of the tea produced in the world is black tea, little research has been done on black tea compared to the number of studies that have been done on green tea. So it is possible that black tea, and maybe all tea, is even healthier than has been thought up to now.

I like the convenience so I'm interested in supplements. I also like the convenience of instant tea. Am I still getting the benefits of the flavonoids?

Sorry. Instant teas and bottled teas only have a fraction of the flavonoids, if they have any at all, of freshly brewed tea, whether the tea has been brewed from loose-leaf tea or using teabags. Flavonoids are believed to lose their power fairly fast (within a few hours) so it's best to drink freshly brewed tea or tea that has been quickly and recently iced.

If I drink green tea instead of taking the supplements, aren't I also getting some of the daily eight glasses of water I'm supposed to drink?

Yes, though the eight glasses theory is being questioned. Some experts say that the caffeine in the tea requires you to drink more than eight glasses but others say that if you're not thirsty you're getting enough water. The majority of experts, though, agree that at least eight glasses, or 64 ounces, of water are necessary for adequate hydration. Water helps regulate all the systems in our bodies, including our appetites. One University of Utah study determined that dehydration may decrease your body's ability to burn calories—up to 2% a day.

German researchers found that after 14 healthy-weight women drank slightly more than two cups of water, their metabolic rate increased for more than an hour (enough to burn 24 calories). If that's true it's another good reason to continually drink tea throughout the day because tea is, of course, mostly water.

One easy way to determine if you're drinking enough water is to check your urine. If it's dark yellow, drink more water. If it's light yellow or clear, you're doing okay.

I bought a box of green tea diet supplements but they don't look right. Can I send them to the FDA for analysis?

The FDA will not analyze dietary supplements sent in by consumers. They suggest that you contact the manufacturer or pay to have a commercial laboratory do the analysis.

If you think a dietary supplement has caused you to be ill, you should first contact your health provider. He or she can then call an FDA hotline to submit a report. In the event of a serious illness that may be related to a dietary supplement, you should call the FDA at 1-800-FDA-1088.

Does it cost more to make tea or buy supplements?

Generally, the supplements cost more, usually around 20–25 cents per capsule, while a cup of tea can be made at home for pennies. Of course, it depends on your taste in tea and which brand of teabags you are purchasing from the grocery store or which kind of loose leaf tea you are buying from a tea shoppe. When doing the math, remember that you can infuse your tea leaves or teabags several times.

Chapter Seven

It Fights Disease, Too

Since the intent of this book was to focus on the weight loss potential of green tea, we didn't plan to write about the other health benefits, but we found they couldn't, and shouldn't, be ignored. Far more research has been done on green tea's disease-prevention and disease-fighting benefits than has been done on its weight-loss aspects. Entire books have been written about what has been discovered in years of research studies.

In this chapter we will just touch on some of the studies that have been published. Then we will list various diseases and conditions and briefly mention some of the findings related to green tea. It is by no means a complete list. If you're interested in green tea's effect on a specific disease or condition but don't have access to the Internet, ask a librarian to help you find the information.

If you are online, a search engine will find your answers. For example, I typed into Google "Kidney disease and green tea" and in less than a second it provided about 477,000 articles it thought might be useful. The first 20 included an article on the Linus Pauling Institute's (University of Oregon) web site that said "Limited research suggests that tea consumption may be associated with fewer cavities and a slightly lower risk of kidney stones." I'm not sure why they put those two together but it goes on to say, of course, that "more research is needed to confirm these findings." Another was the web site of the American Association of Kidney Patients (AAKP) which, after cautioning kidney patients against using many herbal products says, "Green tea is an example of a herb that confers benefit with low risk." A third web site, the University Health Systems of Eastern Carolina's Drug Guide, cautions, "Do not use green tea without first talking to your doctor if you have kidney disease [it lists several other conditions, too]. Green tea contains large amounts of caffeine and may be problematic..." I spent several minutes trying to get the web site's take on coffee's effect on kidney disease if they thought green tea's caffeine was a problem, but could not find mention of it. My guess (and it's just a guess) is that they believe green tea to be an herb, and they are generally wary about all herbal products.

The fourth of the first 20 Google offerings that I looked at was an abstract of an article published in *Asia Pacific Journal of Clinical Nutrition* in 2002 (Vol. 11 (3), pp. 232–6) which said, "In conclusion, kidney function appears to be improved by green tea catechin supplementation....." That site also offered several other articles on the subject, one of which, "Antioxidants in the prevention of renal [kidney] disease," was published in *Renal Failure* (November, 1999, Vol. 21 (6), pp. 581–91) and said, "...atherosclerosis is an important component of chronic renal diseases. There is a wide choice of foods and drugs that could confer benefit. Supplementation with Vitamins E and C, use of soy protein diets and drinking green tea could be sufficient to confer remarkable improvements."

As you can see, opinions and research differ. How do you know what to believe? There's no easy answer. There are long arguments in journals and whenever researchers meet at conferences or conventions as to whether or not a certain study was done correctly or whether methodologies were flawed, statistics skewed, etc. The bottom line is that no food is safe for everyone, but green tea has been shown to do no harm to the vast majority of people who drink it. There are a very few people who are allergic to tea, and some people are so sensitive to caffeine that even the small amount found in green tea bothers them. As mentioned earlier, some doctors say that people who are taking blood thinners should not drink green tea but others say it's not a problem.

If only half of the studies are proven accurate, green tea's health benefits are stunning. If you have any of the diseases or conditions listed, do your own research. Don't expect your doctor to have all of the answers, especially when it comes to nutrition. We'll discuss this more in Chapter Eight. The following are a tiny sampling of published studies.

Immune System

Jack Bukowski, M.D., a professor at Harvard Medical School and a physician at Brigham and Women's Hospital in Boston, also has a PhD in immunology and is licensed in internal medicine and rheumatology. His credentials are mentioned because he has done a lot of work on tea and its impact on the immune system. Since the immune system has a major effect on how our bodies react to infections, diseases, etc., let's look at his work in more detail.

Dr. Bukowski and his teams have been studying the immune system for over a decade. In a recent speech, he talked about how tumor cells are constantly forming in our bodies and how our immune system continually eliminates them. Without our immune systems' constant vigilance the tumor cells could and would grow into various cancers, and bacteria and viruses would overwhelm us within hours.

When an illness spreads through a family causing one person to become quite ill while another isn't affected, it is because of innate immunity, Dr. Bukowski believes. Innate immunity is not well understood, but is being studied, and answers are emerging as to why the same "bug" can have such different effects on people. If you have strong innate immunity, it will act very quickly against the bug and you will have a lighter case or perhaps not feel ill at all.

Components of innate immunity include human gamma delta T lymphocytes (white blood cells), which are different than the majority of white blood cells in our bodies. They are a first line of defense against a wide variety of bacteria, viruses, parasites, and tumors but many people have less than optimal gamma delta T cell function. One of the molecules that activates gamma delta T cells into action is ethylamine, a component of L-theanine. Huge amounts of L-theanine, an amino acid, are found in tea (black, green and oolong), much more than in any other plant. Smaller quantities are found in apple skins, mushrooms, red wine and cucumbers.

Much of the earlier research had been done in petri dishes and in molecular biology experiments, so the team decided to study tea-drinking in humans. Dr. Bukowski's hypothesis going into the study was that tea drinking could enhance natural immunity in humans by priming gamma delta T cells.

In the human study (which was published in 2003), they chose eleven healthy adults who drank less than one cup of tea per month. Blood was taken from each participant and frozen. Then the participants drank

600 ml (a little over 20 oz) of tea (made from Lipton black teabags steeped in water that had been brought to a boil) each day for a month. Blood was drawn each week from the study subjects as well as from participants in the control group, each of whom drank 600 ml of coffee each day for the month. Based on their analysis, the tea drinkers should have gotten about 200 mg of L-theanine each day. When the team tested the blood, only two of the coffee drinkers had a very mild increase in gamma delta T cells. Seven of the 11 tea drinkers, however, had markedly increased gamma delta T cells each week, up to 500 times in some cases.

They also tested the blood against bacteria and found that after only one week the interferon response to the bacteria was markedly increased, sometimes 15 times more than before the tea drinking. Interferon, a protein that boosts the immune system against viruses and helps to fight cancers, is very important for our bodies. Coffee had no effect on the production of interferon.

They also found that introducing L-theanine as a molecule doesn't do the job. The L-theanine must be taken apart to be effective, which our livers do quite nicely.

Dr. Bukowski came to the conclusion that L-theanine is the first discovered nutrient for the immune system from food. And the food with the most L-theanine is tea.

Diseases and conditions

Allergies

Catechins may be effective in hindering histamines from being released, which may relieve various allergy symptoms.

Alzheimer's

Tests at the University of Newcastle found that memory could be improved and Alzheimer's development may be slowed by green tea. It seems to inhibit the activity of the enzyme acetylcholinesterase (AchE). Green tea also hinders the activity of another enzyme, butyrylcholinesterase (BuChE), which has been found in protein deposits on the brains of Alzheimer's patients. The findings of this research were published in the journal *Phytotherapy Research*.

Blood pressure

A 2004 study showed tea prevented high blood pressure. People who drank two cups a day for at least a year had a 46% decreased chance of developing high blood pressure compared to people who drank no tea. Six or more cups showed a decrease chance of 65%.

A study on rats showed that after drinking tea, the rats had lower blood pressure 24 hours later.

A Chinese study concluded that habitual green or oolong tea drinking for more than a year significantly reduced the risk of developing hypertension.

Bone Density

Three studies showed that drinking tea enhances bone-mineral density. Those who drank 3-5 cups per day had higher bone mineral density than those who did not drink tea.

Drinking tea regularly for years may produce stronger bones. Those who drank tea on a regular basis for 10 or more years had higher bone-mineral density in their spines than those who had not.

Carbohydrates

One study showed that green tea causes carbohydrates to be released slowly, preventing sharp increases in blood-insulin levels.

Cardiovascular / Coronary artery disease

A 2004 Japanese study was performed on a group of people who had angiography or heart catheterization to determine the source of pain. It was found that those who did not have coronary artery disease (their pain was due to some other problem) drank an average of almost six cups of tea per day while those with coronary artery disease drank less than four cups per day on average.

Another 2004 study provided corroboration. The study showed that even one cup of tea increased coronary artery blood flow. Coffee did not.

Green tea was shown to decrease LDL (the "bad") cholesterol and protected white blood cells from DNA damage. After 42 days of drinking two cups per day, participants had an average decrease of LDL from 119 to 106.

Published in January of 2005, a 2004 study showed green tea to be associated with decreased P-selectin (which makes blood platelets sticky). Platelets play a role in blocking coronary arteries and brain arteries, so the less sticky the platelets, the better.

One study looked at the coffee- and tea-drinking habits of 340 men and women who had suffered heart attacks and an equal number who had not had heart attacks. They found that drinking one or more cups of tea a day cut the risk of heart attack by 44 percent compared to those who did not drink tea. Coffee, however, had no effect on reducing the risk of heart attacks.

A Saudi Arabia study involving over 3,000 men and women between the ages of 30 and 70 found that those who drank more than six cups of tea per day had significantly lower coronary heart disease than those who did not drink tea, even after adjusting for age and smoking habits. Researchers also found lower serum cholesterol and triglycerides in those who drank at least six cups of tea.

Dutch researchers found even one to two cups of black tea made a difference. Participants had a 46%

lower risk of severe aortic atherosclerosis. Four cups of tea per day made even more difference—a 69% lower risk.

A small Japanese study asked 10 healthy subjects to eat high-fat meals. One group drank water while the other drank black tea. Following the meal it was found blood flow was stronger in those who drank tea.

Cholesterol

EGCG has been shown to effectively lower LDL cholesterol levels and inhibit the formation of abnormal blood clots that can cause heart attacks and stroke. Another study showed black tea lowered blood lipids 6-10 percent within three weeks in people who drank five cups of tea per day. The study showed no effect on HDL, the good cholesterol.

Cancer

The scientific community now believes that at least 30% and perhaps as much as 70% of all cancers are in some way related to nutrition. EGCG inhibits an enzyme needed for cancer cells to grow and can even kill cancer cells without hurting healthy cells.

Bladder cancer

Green tea extracts were found to slow the growth of bladder cancer cells in lab experiments.

Breast cancer

A Japanese study showed that early-stage breast cancer spreads more slowly in women who drink five or more cups of green tea per day.

Leukemia

Taking a capsule equivalent to 10 cups of green tea per day for five months decreased the amount of virus in the blood of patients with human T-cell leukemia virus Type 1. This virus can lead to leukemia, and many of the patients with this virus have depressed immune systems. Theory: the green tea capsule boosted the immune system to be able to fight the virus.

Mayo Clinic researchers found EGCG killed leukemia cells in 8–10 samples from patients with B-cell Chronic Lymphocytic Leukemia (CLL).

Lung cancer

A 2002 study found that drinking five cups of green tea each day may help lower the chance of developing lung cancer, even in smokers.

Ovarian cancer

A study published in late 2004 in China found consumption of green tea lengthens survival in those suffering the most common ovarian cancer. Women who drank tea lived 1–2 years longer than those who did not drink tea—even if they started drinking tea only after they were diagnosed with the disease. But a May, 2004 study in Australia showed that green tea had no effect on ovarian cancer.

Prostate Cancer

Another study done in China last year showed that those who drank tea had less chance of getting prostate cancer and those who drank the most tea had the least chance of getting prostate cancer.

Italian researchers looked at 62 men with precancerous prostate cells. Thirty percent of the men were expected to develop prostate cancer within a year. For the next year half the men were given a capsule containing 600 mg of green tea extract daily while the others were given a placebo. After one year 30% of the men who had been given the placebos developed prostate cancer while only 3% of those who got the green tea extract developed the disease.

Skin cancer

Cleveland's Case Western Reserve University found that green tea applied to the skin may help prevent skin cancer.

Another Case Western study found that ingredients in white tea can boost the skin's immune cells and protect against sun damage and possibly the stresses that cause skin to age.

Dementia

There is ongoing research on dementia and tea that has not yet been completed but there seems to be a relationship between consumption of flavonoids and the development of dementia. Those with the highest intake of flavonoids appear to have the lowest risk of dementia.

Fungus

EGCG enhanced the activities of anti-fungal agents, so mixing tea antioxidants with anti-fungal medicines allowed patients to take lower doses of anti-fungal medicines (which are toxic). Earlier research showed that having patients ingest tea allowed oncologists to increase doses of chemotherapy.

Gastritis

A UCLA School of Public Health study published in May, 2001 found those who drink green tea have half as much chronic gastritis as nondrinkers.

Infection

In a petri-dish experiment, the catechin EGCG was found to enhance the anti-bacterial capabilities of white blood cells taken from lungs. The white blood cells (which eat bacteria), when mixed with antioxidants, ate more bacteria than the white blood cells by themselves. This was true for the lung cells of smokers, too.

Oral health

A study published in early 2005 reported that DNA damage to oral cells in smokers was drastically decreased by the intake of green tea. This is important because DNA damage of oral cells can lead to oral cancer.

Green tea (which naturally contains fluoride) has been shown to destroy bacteria in the mouth. Reports suggest that rinsing with green tea may inhibit cavity- and gum disease-causing bacteria.

Prostatitis

Inflammation of the prostate gland affects almost 30 million men in the United States. It is usually treated with antibiotics, often with little success. A California study indicated that quercetin, another ingredient in green tea, may help men suffering from this painful condition.

Rheumatoid arthritis

Case Western Reserve published a study in 1999 that reported drinking four or more cups of green tea per day may prevent rheumatoid arthritis and reduce its severity in people who already have the disease.

Tea-drinking older women are 60 percent less likely to develop rheumatoid arthritis than those who do not drink tea.

An entire book could be written on the studies that have been published in the last three years on green tea and its effects on various diseases and conditions. It's exciting to see what comes out with each publication. But why wait? Drink tea to lose weight, but also to keep your immune system healthy and to fight disease.

Chapter Eight

What's Right for You?

How much tea do you need to drink each day or how many supplements should you take? In the University of Geneva study discussed in Chapter One, the participants who lost the most weight were given supplements containing 180 mg of EGCG and 100 mg of caffeine each day. That would equal anywhere from one cup to more than six cups of freshly brewed green tea, according to a study published *in Nutrition and Cancer.* Susanne Henning and others from the UCLA Center for Human Nutrition compared the EGCG amounts in eight different brands or kinds of green teabags purchased from local supermarkets and found anywhere from less than 21 mg to more than 99 mg of EGCG when each was infused into 100 ml (less than 1/2 cup) of water.

Since the brewing method was identical for each, it is thought that the disparity could be due to growing conditions and processing methods as well as packaging and storage. As we've already discussed, brewing methods at home can also affect the quality of the tea.

The biggest problem with so much of the research is the lack of standardization in green tea and green tea extracts. Because of the natural differences (geography, climate, soil conditions, etc.) in tea plants as well as the variety of processing procedures and brewing methods, not all brewed tea that is used in research studies is comparable. Extracts can be more standardized but as of this writing, most of them are not. Until all researchers use the same tea compounds, it's difficult to know which studies are more reliable. That may be why we get divergent results such as the following:

- Men who drank ten cups of green tea per day stayed cancer-free three years longer than men who drank fewer than three cups per day.

- Cleveland Western Reserve University studies concluded that drinking four or more cups of green tea per day could help prevent rheumatoid arthritis or reduce the symptoms of the disease.

- Saitama Cancer Research Institute (Japan) discovered fewer recurrences of breast cancer, and the disease spread less quickly, in women with a history of drinking five cups or more of green tea daily.

- A University of California study concluded you could probably get the desired level of polyphenols by drinking two cups per day.

- Great Britain has launched a campaign called "tea4health," encouraging people, especially young people, to drink four cups of tea each day.

Other studies recommend anywhere from one to ten or more cups per day. So back to the question: How much tea should you drink and/or should you take supplements? It's up to you. After all of the research I've done for this book, I've concluded that my goal is to drink no fewer than five cups of tea each day. That's five 8-oz. cups or 40 ounces. I've also decided to take one or two green tea supplements (300 mg with 150 mg polyphenols) each day, which is a major commitment for me because I don't like to take medicine of any sort. However, I do believe the benefits of green tea, whether for weight loss or disease prevention, warrant the effort.

Some people find they don't like the taste of green tea, or any tea. I've found I like white tea a little better than most green teas. I've also made some wonderful combinations of green tea and herbal tisanes, for example, green tea with spicy orange or cinnamon apple. The TeaSource, my favorite tea store in the Twin Cities, makes a chai tea (tea with spices) that is truly a great treat. See Resources for more information.

Marketers are aware that not everyone likes tea, but they also know that everyone wants to be healthy and the majority of us want to lose a few pounds. They are racing each other to come up with a product that will taste good to almost everyone and provide all of the weight-loss-disease-prevention-disease-fighting benefits that green tea has to offer, the "magic" pill or potion. It's undoubtedly a matter of "when," not "if." Until that time, whether it's tomorrow, next year, or 2047, we each have to decide what we want to do now. Unfortunately, your doctor probably won't be able to help you make that decision.

Why don't doctors know more about green tea?

The results of studies on green tea seem to come out weekly, sometimes even daily. Many are ambiguous. That's part of the reason why we don't hear the American Medical Association (AMA) promote the use of green tea. Most doctors, in turn, are hesitant to recommend anything that the AMA hasn't approved. While some results stand the test of time and duplicated studies, others are poorly done and their results are meaningless. Not all scientists and researchers have equal skills, equipment or resources. Some may have personal and/or economic biases (e.g., they may be paid to find the results a company wants them to find). In recent years many journals mention who paid for the studies. Just because a company with a vested interest in the results paid for the research doesn't necessarily mean the study is biased, but it doesn't mean it isn't. Determining the validity of any study is difficult and time consuming.

Most of the time the media have no way of knowing which studies are flawed. Nevertheless, they often report the results (even race each other to report on the study) before others in the scientific community have had time to analyze the quality of the research. So even if a study is reported in the *New York Times* or on CNN, make sure your skeptical antennae are gathering data. And just because the government has approved a drug doesn't necessarily mean it is safe to use.

As we've seen in the last few years, even drugs approved by the FDA and used for years by millions of people have been found to be potentially lethal. The 2004 FDA decision to pull Vioxx off the market is a case in point.

Why do we get such mixed messages? The Mayo Clinic's Brooks Edwards, M.D., explains it best. "Clinical trials are difficult to perform. They yield complicated results that defy straightforward interpretation." He goes on to say that we should first look at who participated in a study and how that group of people relates to us. If it's a group of 25-year-old men and you're a 55-year-old woman, would the results be relevant to you? It's one of the questions you should ask your doctor any time you're prescribed an unfamiliar drug. Something else to talk about with your doctor is the risk/benefit analysis. Know the risks (and all drugs have risks), then ask about the benefits before you decide what to do.

Can't imagine asking your doctor such questions? Is he or she so intimidating or in so much of a rush during your office visit that you would feel uncomfortable questioning his or her recommendations? Don't be. Remember, you're the customer.

At the same time, also remember your doctor is only human. There is so much research to read and so many options for treatment; no doctor can keep up with it all. Doctors often recommend treatments they are most familiar with or have been trained in. That's why surgeons often think the answer is surgery and internal medicine physicians will prescribe a pill rather than a diet change, massage therapy or acupuncture.

Very little nutrition is taught in medical school so don't expect your doctor to know much beyond the basics when it comes to food. In their defense, doctors have a huge workload in medical school and nutrition is often put on the back burner. Your doctor may not be comfortable talking about nutrition or may just give you a standard handout of a low-fat diet. In 1998, according to the Centers for Disease Control (CDC), well over half of American adults were overweight and one-third of that group were obese. At the same time the CDC found that fewer than 10 per cent of doctors even discussed weight loss with patients during office visits.

Some doctors are deciding to take additional coursework on nutrition and even on Eastern philosophies and practices. However, if your doctor is not one of them, you still have alternatives. Integrative medicine is a term that has been used by Dr. Andrew Weil and others who realize that Western medical traditions do not have all the answers and who are willing to explore the wisdom of alternative therapies. The number of doctors practicing integrative medicine is increasing throughout the country. There are also alternative health practitioners, acupuncturists and nutritionists who can help you.

"Medical school doesn't prepare doctors for women patients," says Lila A. Wallis, M.D., clinical professor of medicine at New York's Cornell University Medical College. "Historically, women have not been treated kindly by the established medical profession, as health-care consumers, as health-care providers or as subjects of medical research." In fact, most of the studies that form the foundation of modern medical practice were performed on men. Until 1988, clinical trials of new drugs conducted under the auspices of the FDA were mostly performed on men, though 80% of prescriptions written by doctors were for women. In 1990, Congress provided funding to create the Office of Research on Women's Health with the National Institutes of Medicine.

Why is this important? Here's one example: When researchers got around to looking, they discovered that acetaminophen (Tylenol) is eliminated by women's bodies at about 60% the rate that men eliminate it. Yet prescribed dosages are the same for men and women, which could lead to overdose in women.

Only recently has it been discovered that heart attack symptoms differ between men and women. We also know now that more women than men die each year from heart-related illnesses, but many doctors still don't automatically think, or test for, heart problems when women complain of shoulder pain, weakness, or fatigue without chest pain, all symptoms of a heart attack. As a result, women are less likely to receive the prompt treatment needed.

Whom can you trust? Who knows you best? Who has your best interest in mind? You.

Become an MD—A "Me Doctor"

Being your own doctor means more than just knowing your cholesterol and blood pressure numbers. First and foremost, you have to be honest with yourself, both as your doctor and your patient. That involves taking a really good look at yourself. It's one thing to fudge your weight on your driver's license; it's another to be dishonest with yourself.

It may be even worse not to know. Too many of us are so involved with our careers and/or in taking care of others that we've lost sight of our own health problems, at least until we encounter them the hard way, through a stroke, heart attack or disease. Others of us hate to go to the doctor, fearing what we may hear. Many men hate the idea of prostate testing so much that they simply refuse to have a physical exam.

Before you go to the doctor, take a long, honest look in the mirror. Then find out what your numbers are. Not just your weight but also your body mass index, your blood pressure, your cholesterol numbers, your normal resting pulse, etc. As important as the numbers are, though, they will be meaningless unless you know what they are telling you. If your "other" doctor doesn't explain it clearly, find out for yourself. There are many good family medical books available (a few are listed in the Resource section) that clearly explain what all the numbers mean. Many of them have sections of symptoms, too. Having a reference book on hand can tell you when not to worry as well as when it's necessary to take more action. The Internet, of course, can overwhelm you with data, but it can also be a great resource for more timely information.

Still more

In the pages that follow you'll find even more about tea, including how to recycle your tea leaves and teabags, and how to remove tea stains if you don't recycle them fast enough. There's also a section of tips to assist your green tea weight loss program. In the References section you'll find the research studies I've read, should you want to read them too. And there's a list of resources, books, magazines and web sites I've found particularly helpful or interesting.

I said in the Introduction that I was skeptical about the weight-loss claims for green tea. No longer. I've lost weight. She-who-has-no-asterisk has continued to lose weight too. I feel better than I did before I started drinking green tea and I'd like to hear if it works for you. Please let me know. In the meantime, my teakettle is whistling.

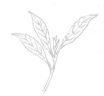

Reuse and Recycle

Whether you use teabags or loose tea, there are many uses for tea around the house and garden. And, of course, you'll need to know what to do about that occasional tea stain. Here's an assortment of tips.

In the kitchen

- Add fresh or used tea leaves to soups, stews, roasts, and other dishes. Sprinkle some in omelets.

- Tea is a natural tenderizer. Use it as a marinade for red meats, chicken, or even tofu.

- Grind tea leaves in a pepper mill, combine with other spices and use as a rub for meat.

- Used teabags or tea leaves can be placed in a small, uncovered bowl to absorb refrigerator odors.

- Wet tea leaves are a natural deodorizer. Rub your hands with them to get rid of fish or garlic odors.

Cosmetic and medicinal uses

- Refresh tired eyes by placing cooled green teabags over each eye for a few minutes.

- Chew a few tea leaves to freshen your breath. Or, one cup of green tea combined with a quart of spring water makes a refreshing mouthwash.

- Add a cup or two of tea to your bath water and allow it to freshen your skin—try green tea with mint. Be sure to rinse thoroughly.

- Crushed fresh tea leaves added to cold cream or another facial cleanser can help slough off old skin. If you use it on your face, gently massage with the cleanser, then rinse.

- Tea's astringency can be useful as an aftershave splash.

- To freshen your feet, soak them in a pan of warm tea water. The anti-fungal properties of tea will help keep your feet healthier, too.

- Used tea leaves that have been allowed to dry can be made into sachets and placed into shoes and boots to absorb moisture and odors.

- Cloth soaked in green tea and placed on sunburned skin will offer immediate comfort. Refrigerated used teabags gently rubbed on the skin will also help. This also helps skin attacked by poison ivy.

- You can also save used teabags, put one in each section of an ice-cube tray. When the tray is full, add water and freeze. The next time you have a bump or bruise, or a razor- or papercut, pull out a tea cube to soothe and heal.

- Eye infections in people and animals can be soothed with a tea-soaked cloth or a used teabag.

- Black tea can be used to halt bleeding after a tooth is extracted; bite down gently on a wet teabag.

- Wet tea leaves can be pressed around a tooth for temporary relief of a toothache.

General cleaning

- Sprinkle dried tea leaves, fresh or used, on a rug or carpet, crush them into the fibers (the kids will love helping with this), wait an hour or so, then vacuum thoroughly. The carpeting will smell fresher and it's easier on the vacuum than baking soda.

- Added to kitty litter, tea leaves can help absorb odors.

Plants and gardening

- Leftover green tea can be used to water plants; the tea leaves, when put on top of the soil of the houseplants, become a mini-compost pile, providing rich nutrients.

- Used tea leaves can be used on outdoor plants, too. Hydrangeas and azaleas especially appreciate tea compost.

- Finally, leaves and bags, minus the tags and staples, can be added to your compost pile.

Natural Dyeing

- Black tea has been used for centuries to dye fabrics, to "antique" them, changing whites into soft ecru shades. Green tea can be used to dye light fabrics into shades of sage green; the strength of the tint will depend on how long the fabric is left in the tea water.

Tea Stains

- For fresh tea stains on fabric, first blot or sponge the spot or spots with cool water. Then stretch the stained fabric over a bowl with the stain side down. Secure it with rubber bands (you could also try an embroidery hoop to hold the fabric taut). Place the bowl and fabric in the bathtub, shower or deep sink and pour boiling water over it from a height of 2–3 feet. Please be careful! If that doesn't work or you want a slightly less dangerous method, try soaking the fabric in a solution of one part vinegar and two parts water, then laundering as usual. Be sure to check the fabric before it goes through a cold rinse cycle to see if you need to work on the stain some more, and definitely before it goes into the dryer. Once it's gone through the dryer, the stain may be set. If that happens, try the vinegar/water solution followed by laundering with an enzyme detergent. Hanging the fabric in the sun may help.

- For tea stains on carpeting, first blot with paper towels to remove as much as possible. Then fill a spray bottle with a mixture of 1/3 cup of white vinegar and 2/3 cup of water. Spray enough to saturate the stained area, then blot again. Is the stain still there? Try a little dishwashing liquid (not the kind for the dishwasher and one that does not contain bleach). Spray it on and blot again. Be sure to rinse the area once the stain is gone and blot to remove most of the water. If the detergent doesn't remove the stain you can try a 3% hydrogen peroxide solution, but first call your carpet's manufacturer or check their web site for additional help. Once the stain is removed you may want to add several layers of paper towels and weigh them down for a few hours to absorb as much water as possible before air drying.

- Tea stains can be removed from teacups and teapots by rubbing with salt, then washing and drying as usual. Or try dipping a damp sponge in baking soda, then rubbing the stain.

- An alternative for teapots: Add 2–3 tablespoons of baking soda or cream of tartar to the teapot. Add boiling water. When it is cool enough scrub the inside of the teapot.

- A paste of baking soda and water will take out any stain left by a teabag on a kitchen counter.

Other Weight Loss Suggestions

Out of sight, out of mind. Ever found yourself not even thinking about food until you try to walk past an open bag of potato chips? Tell everyone in your family to put the food away, far away, so it's not a temptation.

Fish is good for you, right? Not fried fish. Frying apparently alters the protective benefits of fish, the ratio of good to bad fats, and may lead to blood clot formation. Also, don't forget the mercury in many fish. Most doctors recommend that a pregnant woman stay away from canned tuna throughout her pregnancy and while nursing. The rest of us should probably limit our tuna salad to no more than once or twice a week at most.

Sugar is sugar is sugar, whether it's the white kind or the fruit juice kind. And some fruit juices have added sugar! It's better to eat an orange than to drink orange juice because you're getting fiber as well as better quality vitamins and minerals. Got to have juice? Try hand-squeezed, or get the carton of juice with "lots of pulp." Try diluting the juice with sparkling water—no added calories, a "lighter" drink and more thirst-quenching.

Watch your portion sizes

The new Food Pyramid emphasizes portion control, and recent media attention has focused on the supersizing of restaurant portions. Remember, the calories listed on packages are per serving, and your idea of a serving may be very different from that of the manufacturer.

For example:

1 oz. of bread is about the size of an index card.

1 oz. of cheese equals the size of two dice.

3 oz. of meat is about the size of a deck of cards.

One serving of pasta is about the size of a hockey puck.

Another way to judge portions is to use your hand. For example an average-sized woman's hand can be used for the following equivalencies:

Your thumb is roughly equal to one ounce or one tablespoon.

The tip of your thumb is equal to about a teaspoon.

The palm area is about the size of one 3-oz serving of meat, fish or poultry.

To be really sure, try measuring various weights of food and see how they compare to your hand size. If you've already been caught staring at the steam (see Chapter Three) you may want to do this in private. Your children may think you're a little nuts. And speaking of nuts, one handful is one serving of nuts.

Do you think those portions seem awfully small? I did. Another thing I was curious about was plate sizes. When I got out my mother's china (circa 1950s) I noticed the dinner plates seemed quite small. I even wondered if they were the salad plates and I had misplaced the dinner plates. Then I noticed the plates in my mother-in-law's china set were also "small," about eight inches in diameter. The mystery was solved when I heard a nutritionist on the radio say that dinner plates have gotten bigger in the last few decades. They went from 8 inches to 10 inches, and now an average dinner plate is 11 inches or larger. A full dinner plate of that size will hold a lot of food. Try putting your "official serving sizes" of food on a smaller plate.

Spice it up

Foods with capsaicin, which is found in chilies, some mustards, and jalapeno, cayenne and other spicy peppers, have also been found to speed up metabolism, so if you can handle the heat, spice up your meals.

Keep moving

Lost the remote control for the television? Good. Find yourself fidgeting in a meeting? Great. The Mayo Clinic studied 20 individuals (10 lean and 10 obese), all of whom declared themselves to be couch potatoes. Using sensors embedded in special underwear, scientists monitored the movements of the 10 men and 10 women every half-second for 10 days to measure their non-exercise activity thermogenesis (NEAT). In other words, they measured their every movement. Doctors discovered that the lean men and women had a natural propensity to move, even after gaining weight, while the obese were more likely to sit still, even after losing weight. The differences in movement (e.g., standing, walking and, yes, fidgeting) added up to 350 calories per day.

So get up to change the channels, go shopping instead of watching television, put the printer several feet away from your computer so you have to get up to get the printout, play piano. Look for ways to make yourself move if you're one who is more inclined to sit. Those 350 daily calories add up to several pounds each year. More details about the study can be found on the Mayo Clinic web site (www.mayoclinic.org/spotlight/fidget-low-metabolism.html) or the January 29, 2005 issue of *Science* magazine.

Get enough sleep

There's been a lot written lately about sleep and weight loss. Lack of sleep can be a serious problem that is not always easily solved, especially if you have small children or you're going through menopause. Often, though, we're sleep deprived because of television, stress, or any number of reasons that are more-or-less within our control. Studies have shown that when we don't get enough sleep we try to find energy in food. So have a talk with yourself. Is that rerun of *Law and Order* really worth the calories that will tempt you the next day?

Some research has shown L-theanine (which is abundant in tea) promotes relaxation. If you're having trouble getting to sleep, try drinking white tea (it has the least caffeine). It may help more than an over-the-counter sleeping pill and is safer.

Drink more water

I'm learning to drink more water. In her wonderful book, *French Women Don't Get Fat*, Mereille Guiliano writes that French women drink far more water than Americans. She reminds us that our bodies are constantly losing water, even as we sleep, through breathing and perspiration as well as in the more obvious ways. That water should be continually replaced, starting with a full glass of water first thing in the morning. I've tried drinking more water and I have to admit that I can feel the difference the next day when I've had my requisite amount of water the day before. Caffeine is a diuretic so if you drink a lot of tea, especially black tea, or coffee, drink even more water. Green tea, since it has far less caffeine, is the better choice, of course.

Guiliano also points out that we often mistake thirst for hunger. We end up having a snack when what our bodies are craving is water. Fruits and vegetables supply part of the water, but there's not much in a Snickers bar. So the next time you've got the mid-morning munchies, drink a glass of water or have a cup of tea, then allow a few minutes to see if you feel better. If you're still hungry, eat a piece of fruit.

Finally, don't forget to include green tea as an important part of your new, healthy routine.

Resources

Books

Chow, Kit and Ione Kramer. *All the Tea in China.* San Francisco: China Books and Periodicals, Inc., 1990.

Dunford, Marie. *Nutrition Logic: Food First, Supplements Second.* Pink Robin Publishing, 2003.

Guiliano, Mireille. *French Women Don't Get Fat.* New York: Alfred A. Knopf, 2005.

Koop, C. Everett, and the editors of Time Inc Health. *Dr. Koop's Self-Care Advisor: the Essential Home Health Guide for You and Your Family.* New York: Time Inc Health (Time Warner Inc), 1996.

Mitscher, Lester A. and Victoria Dolby. *The Green Tea Book.* New York: Avery (Putnam), 1998.

Perry, Sara. *The New Tea Book.* San Francisco: Chronicle Books, 2001.

Pettigrew, Jane. *The New Tea Companion.* London: National Trust Enterprises Ltd, 2005.

Pratt, Steven and Kathy Matthews. *SuperFoods Rx.* New York: William Morrow (HarperCollins Publishers), 2004.

Roizen, Michael F. and Mehmet C. Oz. *You, the Owner's Manual.* New York: HarperResource (HarperCollins Publishers), 2005.

Rosen, Diana. *The Book of Green Tea.* North Adams, MA: Storey Books, 1998.

Shrader, Carl E. *How To Be Your Own Doctor.* Phoenix: Acacia Publishing, Inc., 2004.

Tokunaga, Mutsuko. *New Tastes in Green Tea.* Tokyo: Kodansha International, 2001.

Magazines

The Tea Magazine, published quarterly by Olde English Tea Company, Inc., 3 Devotion Road, PO Box 348, Scotland, CT 06264. Web site: www.teamag.com

Tea Time, published bimonthly by Hoffman Media LLC, 1900 International Park Drive, Suite 50, Birmingham, AL 35243. Web site: www.teatimemagazine.com

Fine teas and accessories

Elmwood Inn Fine Teas
205 East 4th Street
Perryville, KY 40468
800-765-2139
www.elmwoodinn.com

Harney & Sons Fine Teas
PO Box 665
Salisbury, CT 06068
888-427-6398
www.harney.com

TeaSource
752 Cleveland Ave South
St. Paul, MN 55116
        and
2908 Pentagon Dr NE
St Anthony, MN 55418
877-768-7233
www.teasource.com

Useful web sites

American Association of Kidney Patients
www.aakp.org

Center for Disease Control
www.cdc.gov

Celestial Seasonings Tea
www.celestialseasonings.com

Ceylon Teas
www.ceylon-tea.com

Davidson Teas
www.davidsontea.com

Eastern Tea
www.easterntea.com

English Tea Store
www.englishteastore.com

Dr. Andrew Weil
www.drweil.com

Food and Drug Administration
www.fda.gov

Generation Tea
www.generationtea.com

Gray-Seddon Tea
www.gray-seddon-tea.com

Green Tea Lovers
www.greentealovers.com

In Pursuit of Tea
www.inpursuitoftea.com

Life Extension
www.lef.org

Lipton Tea
www.lipton.com

Linus Pauling Institute
www.lpi.oregonstate.edu

MD Anderson Cancer Center
www.cancerwise.org

MedicineNet
www.medicinenet.com

Mrs. Kelly's Tea
www.mrskellystea.com

Multinational Monitor
www.multinationalmonitor.org

MyWebMD
www.mywebmd.com

National Cancer Institute
www.cancer.gov

Obesity. org
www.obesity.org

Planet Tea
www.planet-tea.com

Serendipitea
www.serendipitea.com

Stash Tea
www.stashtea.com

Tazo Tea
www.tazo.com

Tea Council of Canada
www.tea.ca

Tea Muse
www.teamuse.com

Twinings Tea
www.twinings.com

Unilever
www.unilever.com

Selected bibliography

Chapter 1:

Ashida, Hitoshi. "Anti-obesity actions of green tea: Possible involvements in modulation of the glucose uptake system and suppression of the adipogenesis-related transcription factors." *Biofactors*, 22:135-140, 2004.

Blumberg, Jeffrey. "Introduction to the Proceedings of the Third International Scientific Symposium on Tea and Human Health." American Society for Nutritional Sciences; *Journal of Nutrition*, 133:3244S-3246S, October, 2003.

Chan, Ping Tan et al. "Jasmine green tea epicatechins are hypolipidemic in hamsters (*Mesocricetus auratus*) fed a high fat diet." *Journal of Nutrition*, 129:1094-1101, 1999.

Choo, J. J. "Green tea reduces body fat accretion caused by high-fat diet in rats through adreno-ceptor activation of thermogenesis in brown adipose tissue." *Journal of Nutritional Biochemistry*, 14(11):671. [Abstract]

Dulloo, Abdul et al. "Efficacy of a green tea extract rich in catechin polyphenols and caffeine in increasing 24-hour energy expenditure and fat oxidation in humans." *American Journal of Clinical Nutrition*, 70(6):1040-1045; December, 1999.

Dulloo, Abdul et al. "Green tea and thermogenesis: interactions between catechin-polyphenols, caffeine and sympathetic activity." *International Journal of Obesity*, 24:252-258, 2000.

Dulloo, Abdul G. Letter to the editor: "Reply to Y-H Kao et al." *American Society for Clinical Nutrition*, 7(5): 1233-1234, November, 2000.

Mochizuki, Miyako and Noboru Hasegawa. "Effects of green tea catechin-induced lipolysis on cytosol glycerol content in differentiated 3T3-L1 cells." *Phytotherapy Research*, 18(11):945-946. [Abstract]

Nagao, T. et al. "Ingestion of a tea rich in catechins leads to a reduction in body fat and malondialehyde-modified LDL in men." *American Journal of Clinical Nutrition*, 81(1)122-9, January, 2005.

Wu, Chih-Hsing et al. "Relationship among habitual tea consumption, percent body fat, and body fat distribution." *Obesity Research*, 11:1088-1095, 2003.

Yang, C. S. et al. "Blood and urine levels in tea catechins after ingestion of different amounts of green tea by human volunteers." *Cancer Epidemiology Biomarkers & Prevention*, 7(4):351-354, 1998.

Chapter 2:

Pettigrew, Jane and Bruce Richardson. *The New Tea Companion.* London: National Trust Enterprises Ltd, 2005.

Rosen, Diana. *The Book of Green Tea.* North Adams, MA: Storey Books, 1998.

Chapter 3:

Rosen, Diana. "Iced tea: an American beverage." *Tea Muse,* June 2001. http://www.teamuse.com/article_010602.html

Smith, Steven and Steven L. Wright. "Iced tea: the distinctively American beverage." Tea Association of the United States. http://www.teausa.com/general/icedtea.cfm

Waddington, Bill. "Preparing tea." TeaSource, 2004; www.teasource.com

Chapter 4:

American Dietetic Association. "Position of the American Dietetic Association: functional foods." *Journal of the American Dietetic Association,* 99(10):1278-1285; October, 1999.

American Dietetic Association. "Position of the American Dietetic Association: phytochemicals and functional foods." *Journal of the American Dietetic Association,* 95:493, 1995 (reaffirmed in 1997).

Chen, Z. Y. et al. "Comparison of antioxidant activity and bioavailability of tea epicatechins with their epimers." *British Journal of Nutrition*, 91(6):873-881; June 2004. [Abstract]

Crespy, V. and G. Williamson. "A review of the health effects of green tea catechins in *in vivo* animal models." *Journal of Nutrition*, 134 (12 Suppl): 3432S-3440S; December, 2004. [Abstract]

Challem, Jack. "Antioxidant." *Alternative Medicine*; March, 2005.

Graham, H. N. "Green tea composition, consumption, and polyphenol chemistry." *Preventive Medicine*, 21(3):334-50; May, 1992.

Kroon, Paul and Gary Williamson. "Polyphenols: dietary components with established benefits to health?" *Journal of Science and Food Agriculture*, 85:1239-1240; 2005.

Linus Pauling Institute, Micronutrient Information Center. "Tea." http://lpi.oregonstate.edu/infocenter/ phytochemicals/tea/

Time magazine. "10 foods that pack a wallop." January 21, 2002. http://www.time.com/time/archive/ preview/0, 10987,1001676,00.html

Chapter 5:

Fortier, I., S. Marcoux and L. Beaulac-Baillargeon. "Relation of caffeine intake during pregnancy to

intrauterine growth retardation and preterm birth."
American Journal of Epidemiology, 137(9):931-940;
1993.

Grounds for Change. "Swiss Water Process Decaffeination." http://www.groundsforchange.com/
learn/swiss.php

Mayo Clinic staff. "The caffeine question: Should you
decaffeinate your diet?" http://mayoclinic.com/
invoke.cfm?objectid=62AE24BC-7395-4CF6-
9ADD5159CDA5A865

Mayo Clinic staff. "Miscarriage." http://www.mayo-
clinic.com/invoke.cfm?objectid=5BDD739C-4068-
44CC-AA68C42A79116B33

Reid, T. R., "Caffeine." http://magma.nationalgeo-
graphic.com/ngm/0501/feature1/

Infante-Rivard, C. "Fetal loss associated with caffeine
intake before and during pregnancy." *Journal of the
American Medical Association*, 270(24):2940-3;
December 22-29, 1993.

Pepsi Cola. "What's in Diet Pepsi?" http://www.pepsi-
cola.com/pepsi_brands/product_info/dietpepsi/
index.php

Rhodes, Felisha L. and Donna McDuffie. "Caffeine in
soda and other beverages." University of Minnesota
Extension Service. http://www.extension.umn.edu/
info-u/nutrition/BJ884.html

Whole Foods. "How is tea decaffeinated?" http://www.wholefoods.com/healthinfo/decaftea.html

Yang, Bill. "Caffeine and Health." http://www.2coca-cola.com/ourcompany/columns_caffeine.html

Chapter 6:

Anderson, J. and L. Young. "Weight loss products and programs." Colorado State University Cooperative Extension. http://www.ext.colostate.edu/pubs/foodnut/09363.html

Chen, Z., Q.Y. Zhu, D. Tsang, and Y. Huang. "Degradation of green tea catechins in tea drinks." *Journal of Agriculture and Food Chemistry*, 49(1):477-82; Jan., 2001.

Henning, Susanne M. et al. "Bioavailability and antioxidant activity of tea flavanols after consumption of green tea, black tea, or a green tea extract supplement." *American Journal of Clinical Nutrition*, 80(6):1558-1564; December, 2004.

Lichtenstein, M. D. et al. "Get antioxidants from food, not supplements says American Heart Association." American Heart Association scientific advisory; August 2, 2004. www.americanheart.org/presenter.jhtml?identifier=3023709

MD Anderson Cancer Center. "Mind, body & spirit: being aware of the supplement explosion." *Cancer-Wise*, March, 2003. http://www.cancerwise.org/march-2003

Saper, R.B., Eisenberg, D. M, and R. S. Phillips. "Common dietary supplements for weight loss." *American Family Physician*, 70(9)1731-8; Nov. 1, 2004.

U.S. Food and Drug Administration. "Dietary Supplement Health and Education Act of 1994, Public Law 103-417, 103rd Congress." http://www.fda.gov/opacom/laws/dshea.html

U.S. Food and Drug Administration. "FDA announces major initiatives for dietary supplements." Press release: FDA News; November 4, 2004. http://wwwfda.gov/bbs/topics/news/2004/NEW01120.html

U.S. Food and Drug Administration Center for Food Safety & Applied Nutrition. "Overview of dietary supplements." http://www.csan.fda.gov/!~dms/ds-oview.html; January 3, 2001.

U.S. Food and Drug Administration Center for Food Safety & Applied Nutrition. "Tips for the savvy supplement user: making informed decisions and evaluating information." http://www.cfsan.fda.gov/~dms/ds-savvy.html; January, 2002.

Zhou, Y. D., et al. "Hypoxia-inducible factor-1 activation by (-)-epicatechin gallate: potential adverse effects of cancer chemoprevention with high-dose green tea extracts." *Journal of Natural Products*, 67(12):2063-9; Dec., 2004.

Chapter 7:

Ahmad, Nihal et al. "Green tea constituent Epigallo-catechin-3-Gallate and induction of apoptosis and cell cycle arrest in human carcinoma cells." *Journal of the National Cancer Institute*, 39(24): 1881-1886; December 17, 1997.

Bukowski, J. F., Morita, C. T., and M. B. Brenner. "Human gamma delta T cells recognize alkylamines derived from microbes, edible plants, and tea: implications for innate immunity." *Immunity*, 11(1):57-65; 1999.

Bukowski, Jack. "Interview with Jack Bukowski, MD. Topic: The impact of *Camelia Sinensis* (Tea) on hearing." *Healthy Hearing*, June 9, 2003. http://www.healthyhearing.com/healthyhearing/newroot/interview/displayarchives.asp?id=126&catid=1089

Mukhtar, Hasan and Nihal Ahmad. "Tea polyphenols: prevention of cancer and optimizing health." *American Society for Clinical Nutrition*, 7(6):1698s-1702s; June, 2000.

Mukamal, Kenneth J., et al. "Tea consumption and mortality after acute myocardial infarction." *Circulation*, 105:2476; 2002.

Murase, Takatoshi et al. "Green tea extract improves endurance capacity and increases muscle lipid oxidation in mice." *American Journal of Physiology Regulatory, Integrative and Comparative Physiology.*, 228: R708-R715; 2005.

Naasani, Imad et al. "Blocking telomerase by dietary polyphenols is a major mechanism for limiting the growth of human cancer cells *in vitro* and *in vivo.*" *Cancer Research*, 63:824-830; February 15, 2003.

Reaney, Patricia. "Anti-cancer compound in green tea." Reuters report. News.com.au; March 15, 2005.

Riemersma, R. A. et al. "Tea flavonoids and cardiovascular health." *Journal of Medicine*, 94:277-282; 2001.

Wardle, E. N. "Antioxidants in the prevention of renal disease." *Renal Failure*, 21(6):581-91; November, 1999. [Abstract]

Yang, Y. C., et al. "The protective effect of habitual tea consumption on hypertension." *Archives of Internal Medicine*, 164(14):1534-40; July 26, 2004.

Chapter 8:

Benzie, Iris F. F. and Y. T. Szeto. "Total antioxidant capacity of teas by the ferric reducing/antioxidant power assay." *Journal of Agriculture and Food Chemistry*, 47:633-636; 1999.

Henning, Susanne M., et al. "Catechin content of 18 teas and a green tea extract supplement correlates with the antioxidant capacity." *Nutrition and Cancer* 45(2):226-235; 2003.

Khokar, S. and S. G. Magnusdottir. "Total phenol, catechin, and caffeine contents of teas commonly consumed in the United Kingdom." *Journal of*

Agriculture and Food Chemistry, 50(3):565-70; Jan. 30, 2002. [Abstract]

Pratt, Steven and Kathy Matthews. *SuperFoods Rx*. New York: William Morrow (HarperCollins Publishers), 2004.

Additional Resources:

Used in Multiple Chapters or for Background Information:

Books:

Bales, Keith and Gillian. *The Green Tea Lifestyle*. Victoria, B.C.: Trafford, 2004.

Batmanghelidj, F. *Water for Health, For Healing, For Life: You're Not Sick, You're Thirsty!* New York: Warner Books, 2003.

Articles:

Bell, Stacey J. and G. Ken Goodrick. "A functional food product for the management of weight." *Critical Reviews in Food Science and Nutrition*, 43(2)163-178; March-April, 2002. [Abstract]

Chow, H. H. Sherry, et al. "Phase I pharmacokinetic study of tea polyphenols following single-dose administration of Epigallocatechin gallate and Polyphenon E." *Cancer Epidemiology Biomarkers & Prevention*, 10:53-58; January, 2001.

Dalluge, Joseph J. et al. "Capillary liquid chromatography/electrospray mass spectrometry for the separation and detection of catechins in green tea and human plasma." *Rapid Communications in Mass Spectrometry,* 11(16)1753-1756. Published online: 4 Dec. 1998.

Drewnowski, Adam and Carmen Gomez-Carneros. "Bitter taste, phytonutrients, and the consumer: a review." *American Journal of Clinical Nutrition,* 72(6):1424-1435; December, 2000.

Lin, Y. S. et al. "Factors affecting the levels of tea polyphenols and caffeine in tea leaves." *Journal of Agriculture and Food Chemistry,* 51(7):1864-73; March 26, 2003.[Abstract]

McKay, Diane, et al. "The role of tea in human health: an update." *Journal of the American College of Nutrition,* 21(1):1-13; 2002.

Richelle, Myriam, Isabelle Tavazzi and Elizabeth Offord. "Comparison of the antioxidant activity of commonly consumed polyphenolic beverages (coffee, cocoa, and tea) prepared per cup serving." *Journal of Agriculture and Food Chemistry,* 49: 3438-3442; 2001.

Serafini, M., Ghiselli, A. and A. Ferro-Luzzi. "*In vivo* antioxidant effect of green and black tea in man." *European Journal of Clinical Nutrition,* 50(1):28-32; January, 1996.

Yang, Chung S. "Effects of tea consumption on nutrition and health." *Journal of Nutrition*, 130:2409-2412; 2000.

Glossary of Terms

Antioxidant: a substance that blocks or neutralizes free radicals; protects the body against tissue damage.

Black tea: tea that has been fully oxidized; the world's most popular tea.

Bud: the unopened top leaf of a stem of the tea bush.

Caffeine: part of a group of compounds called methyl-xanthines found in leaves and seeds of over 60 plants, including cocoa beans and tea leaves.

***Camellia sinensis*:** botanical Latin name for the tea plant.

Catechins: part of the larger group of antioxidant polyphenols.

Chai tea: chai is the Indian word for tea; today it usually means a tea flavored with milk and several spices.

Dust: the finest particles of tea leaves left remaining after processing. Also called fannings.

Epicatechin (EC): polyphenol catechin antioxidant found in green tea.

Epicatechin gallate (ECG): polyphenol catechin antioxidant found in green tea.

Epigallocatechin (EGC): polyphenol catechin antioxidant found in green tea.

Epigallocatechin gallate (EGCG): The strongest polyphenol catechin antioxidant found in green tea.

Extract: to remove or separate substances by pressure, distillation or evaporation; also, another word for supplement.

Fannings: the finest particles of tea leaves remaining after processing. Also called tea dust.

Fermentation: a term often used when referring to oxidation; the process of enzyme oxidation that changes the color and characteristics of the tea leaf.

First flush: the first tea leaves picked in the new growing season.

Flavonoid: a naturally occurring compound of the polyphenol family; it has antioxidant properties.

Fluoride: a compound naturally found in tea; it prevents tooth decay.

Free radicals: molecules produced by the body that cause disease and aging.

Functional food: term for foods that have health benefits other than vitamins and minerals.

Green tea: tea that has been minimally oxidized, oxidized less than oolong and black tea. Green tea has considerable antioxidants that are thought to prevent and fight disease. It can also increase metabolism and burn fat.

Herbal tea: a beverage made from herbs and not made from the *Camellia sinensis* bush; the correct term is tisane.

Infusion: a liquid product obtained by steeping; the absorption of water.

L-theanine: an amino acid found in tea that may have health benefits.

Metabolism: energy expenditure within the human body.

Nutraceutical: coined from the terms nutrition and pharmaceutical, it is a substance considered to be a food, or part of a food, that provides health benefits.

Obesity: the condition of excessive body fat (more than 20% above the ideal).

Oolong tea: partially oxidized tea; the tea normally served in Chinese restaurants.

Orange pekoe: a grade of tea larger than pekoe; it has nothing to do with oranges.

Oxidation: the chemical change that occurs when oxygen combines with another substance.

Panfire: a method of removing moisture from tea leaves by heating over fire.

Pekoe: a grade of black tea, it includes a bud and two top leaves of a certain size.

Phytochemicals: chemicals found in plants; used to refer to components in plants that have a physiological (antioxidant) effect on humans such as preventing disease or enhancing health.

Phytomedicines: medicines with a plant base.

Phytonutrients: plant-based compounds.

Plucking: the picking of tea leaves.

Polyphenols: antioxidant substances found in tea.

Pu-erh tea: tea made from aged leaves; considered to be a health drink.

Red tea: Chinese reference to black tea; in the U.S. it usually refers to Rooibos tea.

Rooibos: a South African herb shrub, *Aspalathus linearis*. Rooibos is caffeine-free and has many health benefits.

Second flush: the second tea leaves picked in a growing season.

Steep: to soak (tea leaves) in water to extract flavor, catechins and nutrients.

Supplements: vitamins, minerals or other substances in capsule, pill or powder form used to enhance diet.

Tea ball: usually a perforated metal ball to hold tea while it is steeping.

Teabag: a porous sack of various materials used to hold an individual serving of tea leaves.

Thermogenesis: the burning of fat calories.

Tisane: an infused beverage made from herbs and water.

White tea: the least processed tea; it has more anti-oxidants than green tea.

Withering: the removal of moisture from tea leaves to the point of flaccidity.

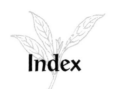

Index

AAKP—See American Association of Kidney Patients
Absorption, 16, 70
Acetaminophen, 61, 106 *See also* Tylenol
Acid reflux, 62
Addiction, caffeine, 61
Afternoon tea, 39
Aftershave, 110
Age, 6, 57, 70, 91, 94
Alkaloid, 59
Allergies, 29, 64, 85, 89
Allergy, caffeine, 64
Alternative health practitioner, 105
Altitude, 20, 22, 66
Alzheimer's, 89
AMA—See American Medical Association
American Association of Kidney Patients, 84

American Classic tea, 28
American Medical Association, 102
Anacin, 60
Anti-fungal, 95, 110
Antioxidant, 7, 10, 11, 13, 24, 55-57, 58, 70, 71, 73, 74, 85, 95
Anxiety, 62, 64
Aortic atherosclerosis, 92
Appetite suppressant, 61
Aroma, 19, 40, 68
Arthritis, rheumatoid, 96, 100
Aspalathus linearis, 28
Aspirin, 61, 75
Asthma, 60
Australia, 19, 23, 28, 94

Bacteria, 25, 50, 51, 56, 86, 87, 88, 95, 96
Barq's Root Beer, 60, 65

Beans, 53
Beer belly, 5
Beta-carotene, 16, 56, 74
Bladder, 62, 92
Bladder cancer, 92
Blood cells, white, 95
Blood clots, 115
Blood platelets, 91
Blood pressure, 12, 61, 89, 107
Blood sugar, 62
Blueberries, 53
Body mass, 63
Body mass index, 14, 107
Boiling water, 29, 36, 41, 43, 44, 68, 112, 114
Bone density, 90
Bottled tea, 80
Bottles
  care of, 51
  metal-lined, 35, 50
  plastic, 35, 37, 50-52
  water, 35, 37, 50-52
Breast cancer, 93, 100
Breast milk, 63
Brewing, 29, 35-45, 47, 48, 66, 67, 99
British teabags, 46
Broccoli, 53
Bubbles, 44
Bukowski, Jack, 86-88

Caffeine, 6, 10, 11, 12, 13, 29, 59-70, 72, 99, 119, 120
  absorption, 67
  allergy, 64
  amounts, 65, 69
  in tea, 66
  in tea extracts, 72
  sensitivity, 63
  withdrawal, 66
Calories, 5, 16, 60, 118
Camellia sinensis, 19, 27
Cancer, 56, 57, 62, 74, 86, 88, 92-94, 96, 100
Cancer treatment, 56
Cancer
  bladder, 92
  breast, 62, 93, 100
  lung, 93
  oral, 96
  ovarian, 74, 93-94
  prostate, 94
  skin, 94
Capsaicin, 117
Carbohydrates, 90
Carbon dioxide, 67, 68
Cardiovascular disease, 12, 15, 90-92
Carpet, 111, 113
Catechin, 10, 13, 14, 16, 17, 54, 55, 58, 67, 68, 71, 74, 85, 89, 95

CDC—See Centers for Disease Control

Centers for Disease Control, 104

Ceylon, 30

Charleston Tea Gardens, 28

Chemicals, 16, 24, 30, 31, 61

Chemotherapy, 56

Chicken soup, 16

China, 19, 20, 25, 26, 29, 30, 93, 94

Chinese restaurants, 27

Chlorine, 36, 37, 45

Chocolate, 54, 65, 66

Cholesterol, 15, 26, 91, 92, 107

   levels, 15, 91, 92

   serum, 15

Chromium, 74

Cleaning, 111

Climate, 20, 21, 100

Clinical trials, 105

Coca-Cola, 60, 64, 65

Coffee, 6, 12, 58, 59, 60, 61, 62, 63, 64, 65, 67, 82, 86, 88, 89, 118, 120

Coffeemaker 47, 48, 49

Colic, 29

Color, 40, 45

Compost, 110-111

Container, 41

Copper, 36

Coronary artery disease, 90-92

Cosmetic uses, 110-111

Cost comparison, 82

Coumadin, 75

Crush, tear, curl, 27

CTC—See Crush, tear, curl

Cuttings, 21

Decaffeinated tea, 12, 62, 65, 67, 68, 69

Decaffeination, 66-68, 69

Decaffeination, do-it-yourself, 68

Dehydration, 81

Dementia, 95

Deodorizer, 109

Diet Coke, 64, 65

Dietary supplement, 55, 75, 76, 78, 82

Dietary Supplement Health and Education Act, 76-78

Digestive organs, 61

Dioxin, 51

Disease prevention, 24, 73, 83

Disease-fighting, 15, 83-97

Distilled water, 37

Diuretic, 61, 120

Doctor, 4, 8, 56, 63, 66, 75, 84, 85, 86, 102, 103, 104, 105, 106, 107, 115, 118

Drinking water, 37

DSHEA—See Dietary Supplement Health and Education Act
Dust, tea, 25, 72
Dyeing fabric, 112
EC—See Epicatechin
ECG—See Epicatechin gallate
EGC—See Epigallocatechin
EGCG—See Epigallocatechin gallate
Eggs, 69-70
Energy expenditure, 10, 11
Enzyme, 17
Epicatechin, 54
Epicatechin gallate, 54
Epigallocatechin, 54, 74
Epigallocatechin gallate, 10, 13, 54, 55, 58, 73, 78, 92, 93, 95, 99
Ethyl acetate, 67
Ethylamine, 87
Excedrin, 60
Exercise, 56
Exercise-induced free radical damage, 56
Extract, green tea, 7, 10, 12, 13, 14, 71-82, 92, 94, 100
Extracts, 71-82, 100 See also Supplements
Eye infections, 111

Fabric, 112
Fabric dyeing, 112
Fair Trade, 32
Fair Trade associations, 32
Fannings, 25, 72
Fat, burning of, 6, 10, 12, 15, 17
FDA—See Food and Drug Administration
Federal Trade Commission, 75-76
Feet, 110
Fiber, 73, 115
Filters, water, 36, 37
First flush, 23
Fish, fried, 115
Flask, 50
Flavanols, 54
Flavonoids, 54, 57, 69, 72, 80
Flavonols, 24, 54, 71
Flavor, 39
Flavoring, 39
Flowers, 25, 45
Fluoride, 36, 96
Food and Drug Administration, 75-78, 82, 103, 105
Food pyramid, 116
Food, functional, 16
Free radicals, 55, 56
Freezer storage, 41
Freezing tea, 41
Freezing teabags, 111

French Women Don't Get Fat, 119
Freshman, 6, 15
Fruit, 39, 55, 56, 115
Fruit juice, 39, 115
FTC—See Federal Trade Commission
Functional foods, 16
Fungus, 95, 110

Gallstones, 61
Gamma delta T lymphocytes, 87-88
Garden plants, 111-112
Gastritis, 95
Gastrointestinal distress, 64
Geography, 23, 100
Ginkgo biloba, 75
Green tea—See Tea, green
Growing conditions, 23, 99
Growing—See Tea, growing
Guiliano, Mereille, 119-120
Gum disease, 96

Hand tremors, 62
Hand, used for measuring, 116-117
Hand-plucking, 21, 22, 23
Hand-processing, 21, 22-24, 29
Hangover, 62
Harvesting, 21, 22, 23
HDL, 92

Headaches, 61, 64, 66
Headaches, migraine, 61
Health benefits, 16, 35, 53, 54, 57, 72, 73, 83, 85
Heart attack, 106
Heart rate, 13
Heartburn, 62
Henning, Susanne, 71, 99
Herb, 84
Herbal products, 79, 84
Herbal tea, 27, 39, 101 *See also* Tisane
Herbicides, 30
Houseplants, 111
Humidity, 41
Hyperfiltration, 37, 89
Hypertension, 12, 89
Iced tea, 48, 49
  invention of, 49
  making, 49
Immune system, 86-88, 93, 97
Immunity, innate, 86-88
India, 29
Infection, 95
Infuser, 44, 45
Infusion, 82
Innate immunity, 86-88
Instant tea, 80
Integrative medicine, 105
Interferon, 88
Internet, 4, 72, 78, 108
Irritability, 66

Kenya, 30
Kidney disease, 83-84, 85
Kidney stones, 84
Kidneys, 61, 83-84, 85
Kitchen tips, 109
Kitty litter, 111

L-theanine, 87, 119
Laxative, 61
LDL, 91
Lead, 36
Leukemia, 93
Linus Pauling Institute, 84
Long-life tea, 29
Loose-leaf tea, 25, 40, 80, 109
Lung cancer, 74, 93-94

Manson, JoAnn, 73
Matthews, Kathy, 53
Me Doctor, 107-108
Measuring tea, 42, 47
Meat rub, 109
Mechanization, 21, 23
Media, 103
Medicinal uses, 110-111
Melaleuca alternifolia, 28
Metabolism, 6, 10, 11, 12, 13, 15, 16, 17, 75, 76, 81, 117
Micronutrients, 53, 54
Microwaving, 47
Middle-age spread, 5, 6

Migraine headaches, 61
Milk, 33, 57
Minerals, 37
Miscarriage, 63
Moderation, 70
Mouthwash, 110
Movement, 118

Nagle, Dan, 74
National Institutes of Medicine, 106
Nausea, 64
NEAT—See Non-exercise activity thermogenesis
Non-exercise activity thermogenesis, 118
Nung, Shen, 19
Nursing infants, 29, 63
Nursing mothers, 63
Nutraceuticals, 16, 53
Nutrients, 6, 53, 57, 70, 73, 88, 99, 111
Nutrition, 4, 77, 86, 92, 104, 105, 106

Oats, 53
Odors, refrigerator, 109
Office of Research on Women's Health, 106
Olympic committee, 60
Oral cancer, 96
Oral health, 96

Oranges, 53
Organic certification, 31
Organic tea, 30-31
Osteoporosis, 61
Ovarian cancer, 74, 93-94
Over-boiling water, 36
Oxidation, 10, 12, 24, 27, 29, 80
Oxygen, 24, 47, 55, 56

P-selectin, 91
Pain relievers, 61
Pan-frying, 24
Parkinson's disease, 60
Pesticides, 30, 31, 79
Physical stress, 63, 70, 94
Physician—See Doctor
Phytochemicals, 16, 73, 80
Phytonutrients, 53, 54-55
Picking (plucking), 21, 22
Plants, garden 111-112
Plastic bottles, 50-52
Plastic bottles, care of, 51
Plates, dinner, 117
Plucking, 21, 22
Plucking plateau, 21
Plucking table, 21
PMS, 61
Poison ivy, 111
Polycarbonate, 51
Polyphenol, 10, 24, 40, 49, 54, 73, 78, 101
Portions, 116-117

Pratt, Steven, 53
Pregnant women, 29, 63, 115
Proanthocyanidins, 54
Processing — See Tea, processing
Processing, orthodox, 24
Processing, traditional, 24
Prostate cancer, 94
Prostate, testing, 107
Prostatitis, 96
Psychological stress, 59, 63, 94, 119
Pu-erh tea—See Tea, Pu-erh
Pulse, 107
Pumpkin, 53

Quercetin, 96

Re-boiling water, 47
Recycling tea, 52
Red bush tea, 28
Red tea, 28 See also Rooibos
Refrigerator odors, 109
Refrigerator storage, 41
Refrigerator temperature, 41
Research, 3, 4, 6, 7, 9, 10, 15, 29, 54, 57, 75, 79, 83, 84, 85, 86, 87
Researchers, 7, 9, 10, 54, 71, 85, 86, 87, 100, 102, 106
Restlessness, 64
Re-using tea, 109-114
Reverse osmosis, 37

Rheumatoid arthritis, 96, 100
Rooibos, 28-29, 39
Root beer, Barq's, 60, 65

Salmon, 53
Saucepan, 44
Scales, 42
Scientists, 9, 102 *See also* Researchers
Second flush, 23
Sensitivity, caffeine, 63
Serum cholesterol, 15, 91
Serum level, 15
Skin cancer, 94
Skin irritation, 29
Skin, sunburned, 110
Sleep, 62, 119
Smallholdings, 21, 24
Smokers, 93, 95, 96
Soil, 20, 23, 31, 66, 100
South Africa, 29
Soy, 53
Spices, 39, 41
Spinach, 53
Spring water—See Water, spring
Sri Lanka, 19, 30
St. Louis Exposition, 48
Stains, tea, 112-114
Standardization, 71, 73, 100
Steam, 44

Steaming of tea leaves, 24
Steeping, 42, 44-45
Stomach upset, 26
Storage, freezer, 41
Storage, refrigerator, 41
Storing tea, 40-42
Stress, physical, 63, 70, 94
Stress, psychological, 59, 63, 94, 119
Studies, validity of, 102
Sugar, 57, 115
Sun tea, 49
Sunburn, 110
Super foods, 53
Superfoods Rx, 53
Supplement Facts, 73, 76, 77
Supplement, safety of, 75, 78
Supplements, 71-82, 101 *See also* extracts
  analyzing, 79, 82
  choosing, 78-80
  claims about, 75, 77
  dietary, 55, 77
  researching, 79

Tap water, 36, 37
Tasters, tea, 30
Tea
  allergies to, 85
  aroma of, 19, 40, 68
  black, 7, 23, 27, 28, 43, 53, 54, 57, 65, 66, 71, 80, 87,

88, 91, 92, 111, 112, 120
bottled, 80
brewing, 35-37, 42-45, 47, 48
buying, 39-40, 42
caffeine in, 65-67
choosing, 39-40
color of, 40, 45
decaffeinated, 12, 62, 65, 67-68, 72
decaffeination of, 67-68
freezing, 41
green, 2, 2-10, 16, 23, 35, 39, 45, 53, 54, 57, 66, 71, 80, 87, 88, 91, 92, 111, 120
and weight loss, 9-17, 57
antioxidant levels, 58
brewing, 42-45, 47-48
health benefits, 73, 85
long-term use, 13
metabolic action, 16
harvesting, 22-23
loose-leaf, 25, 40, 80, 109
growing, 19-22
herbal, 27 See also Tisane
iced, 48, 49, 80
instant, 80
long-life, 29
loose-leaf, 25, 40, 80, 109
measuring, 42, 47
oolong, 14, 23, 27, 87, 89
organic, 30-31

plucking, 22-23
processing, 23, 24-26, 54
Pu-erh, 9, 26
quality of, 46
recycling, 109-112
red, 28 See also Rooibos
red bush, 28
reusing, 109-111
Rooibos, 28-29, 39
steeping, 44-45
storing, 40-42
sun, 49
taste of, 20, 25, 30, 36-37, 39, 41, 42, 43, 46, 47, 50, 57, 101-102
transporting, 50-52
white
antioxidants in, 57
brewing, 29
caffeine in, 65
Tea ball, 45
Tea container, 41
Tea cubes, 49
Tea dust, 25, 72
Tea estates, 19
Tea fannings, 25, 72
Tea gardens, 19
Tea leaves, 11, 20, 21, 22, 23, 24, 25, 35, 40, 41, 42, 45, 47, 49, 67, 68, 69, 80, 82, 108, 109, 110, 111, 112
grading, 25
pan frying, 24

rolling, 25
shaping, 25
sorting, 25
steaming, 24
Tea merchants, 38, 40
Tea plant, 19, 20, 21-22
Tea plantations, 19
Tea press, 47
Tea stains, 112-114
Tea tasters, 30
Tea tree oil, 27
Tea trivia, 33
Tea varieties, 19, 20, 39, 40
Tea workers, 31, 32
Tea workers, wages, 32
Tea4Health, 101
Teabag, 25, 35, 38, 40, 42, 43, 44, 45, 46, 49, 66, 72, 80, 82, 88, 99, 108, 109, 110, 111, 112, 114
British, 46
freezing, 111
freshness of, 40
re-use, 82
Teacups, 35, 113
Teacups, removing stains, 113
Teakettle, 35, 41, 44, 108
Teakettle, whistling, 44, 108
Teapots, 35, 44, 45, 113, 114

Teapots, removing stains, 113, 114
TeaSource, 101, 124
Temperature, refrigerator, 41
Temperature, water, 29, 35, 43, 44, 46, 47, 66, 67
Tenderizer, 109
Theaflavins, 54
Thearubigins, 54
Theine, 69
Thermometer, candy, 43, 47
Thermos, 35, 50
Time magazine, 53, 73
Tips, 33, 109
Tisane, 27, 39, 101
Tomatoes, 53
Tooth decay, 96
Toothache, 111
TransFair USA, 32
Transporting tea, 50-52
Triglycerides, 15, 91
Trimethylxanthine, 59
Trivia, tea, 33
Tuna, 115
Turkey, 53
Tylenol, 61, 106

University of Geneva study, 9-13, 14, 73, 99
Urine, 81

Vacuum flask—See Thermos
Vegetables, 55, 56
Vioxx, 103
Vitamin A, 55, 56
Vitamin C, 55
Vitamin E, 55, 75
Vitamin K, 75
Vitamins, 115

Wadmalaw Island, 28
Wages, 31
Wallis, Lila, 105
Walnuts, 53
Water
  bottles, 35, 37, 50-52
  boiling, 19, 29, 36, 41, 43, 44, 68, 112, 114
  distilled, 37
  drinking, 37, 119-120
  hard, 36
  filters, 36, 37, 49
  microwaving, 47
  re-boiling, 47

spring, 37, 49, 110
tap, 36
taste of, 36-37, 40
temperature, 29, 35, 43, 44, 46, 47, 66, 67
well, 37
Weight loss, 10, 26, 35, 83, 104
Weight-loss claims, 1
Weil, Andrew, 105, 124
Well water, 37
White blood cells, 56, 87, 88, 91, 95
White tea—See Tea, white
Wine, 20, 53, 54, 87
Wine, red, 53, 54, 87
Withdrawal, caffeine, 66
Withering bins, 24
Workers, tea, 31, 32
Working conditions of tea workers, 32
World War II, 33

Yield, 23
Yogurt, 53

Zhou, Yu-Dong, 74

About the Author

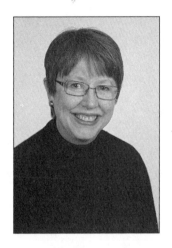

Patricia Rouner, who lives in St. Paul, Minnesota, is co-author of the *New Business Values for Success in The Twenty-first Century* and has edited a wide range of publications: medical textbooks, children's books and sailing magazines. She used green tea to lose the 30 pounds that had mysteriously appeared over the last 30 years.

Order form

Name _____

Address _____

City/State _____ Zip/Postal Code _____

Phone _____ Country (Outside U.S.A) _____

Title	Qty	Price	Total
Lose Weight With Green Tea	____	**$14.95**	____

Shipping: U.S. orders shipped by Media Mail ($4.50 – 1-2 Weeks) or Priority Mail ($6.00 – 1 Week). For UPS rates or bulk orders call 651-490-9408. Canadian orders shipped by Airmail ($7.00)

Total	____
MN residents add sales tax	____
Shipping	____
Total Enclosed (U.S. Funds only)	____

❑ Check   ❑ Money Order   ❑ Visa   ❑ M/C   ❑ Discover   ❑ AMEX

Card # _____ Exp. Date _____

Signature _____

4 Ways To Order

Mail: Box 17948, St. Paul, MN 55117
(check or credit card)

Toll-Free Phone: 1-888-220-5402
(9A.M.–5P.M. CST Monday–Friday, U.S./Canada only)

FAX: 1-651-490-1450

www.SmithHousePress.com